Personal Trials

Personal Trials

How terminally ill ALS patients took medical
treatment into their own hands

Jef Akst

COVER DESIGN BY KERRY ELLIS

Copyright © 2016 Jef Akst
All rights reserved.

ISBN: 1533461554
ISBN 13: 9781533461551
Library of Congress Control Number: 2016908667
CreateSpace Independent Publishing Platform
North Charleston, South Carolina

Contents

Prologue	Death sentence	ix
Chapter 1	Clinical optimism	1
Chapter 2	Learning to live with ALS	5
Chapter 3	Hidden treasure?	16
Chapter 4	An infusion of hope	30
Chapter 5	DIY medicine	40
Chapter 6	On their own	52
Chapter 7	Learning to die	58
Epilogue	Capitalizing on DIY medicine	65
Afterword		73
Author's note		75
Notes		77

Editor's note: All quotes have been taken from direct correspondence or from online forums (permission obtained from these individuals or their families), unless otherwise noted. In some cases, they have been edited for spelling, grammar, and clarity. When sources recalled something they said or thought previously, or what others had told them, quotes are italicized.

Prologue

DEATH SENTENCE

**ERIC VALOR, DIAGNOSED MARCH 2005 AT AGE THIRTY-SIX
SANTA CRUZ, CALIFORNIA**

In early 2004, Eric Valor's left foot started to misbehave. At first he wrote it off as a stretched or torn tendon; he must have injured himself as he ran two at a time down the concrete steps along the side of his Santa Cruz beach cottage, lugging concrete or other construction material to the brick patio he was building. But the problem only got worse. Despite years on a surfboard, he began having trouble timing his drop

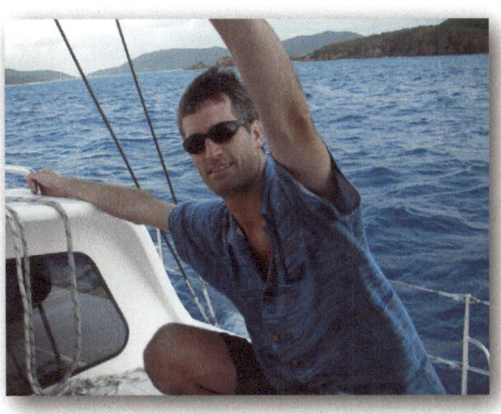

Eric Valor
PHOTO BY CLAIRE VALOR

into a wave. It made for some spectacular wipeouts, and eventually he had to face the fact that something wasn't right. Several months and many doctors later, Eric finally received his answer—and the diagnosis gave him less than five years to live.

Eric looked out the window as he sat with his wife Claire in the office of Dr. Catherine Lomen-Hoerth at the University of California, San Francisco's ALS Center. Ten stories down, he could see runners circling the quarter-mile track and students tossing a Frisbee on the damp football field in the center. It seemed a cruel view given the news he was about to receive: in less than two years he would no longer be able to join them. He would soon lose all the strength in his limbs, and eventually in his throat and diaphragm as well. And the chances were high that, not long after, Claire would be left alone to carry on the life they had started together.

Finally, Dr. Lomen-Hoerth entered. She was young but professional. She sat behind the desk and glanced at Eric's chart one last time, then shifted her gaze to meet his. *Mr. Valor*, she said, *I am afraid the tests indicate amyotrophic lateral sclerosis. There are more tests we can do to try to rule it out, but that is where we are right now.*

His body tensed. ALS, also known as Lou Gehrig's disease, is a slow but relentless deterioration of the motor neurons in the brain stem and spinal cord. Its victims become paralyzed and eventually lose their ability to eat and breathe on their own. There is no effective treatment; there is no cure.

Eric's emotions spread like fire through his body, triggering an explosion of the very power that was already on its way out. His jaw tightened. He had to concentrate to ensure that he did not break Claire's hand with his powerful grip. "My mind alternated between escape, plans to complete life goals in the remaining time, and how I was going to set Claire up for life after me," Eric wrote in his unpublished memoir. "My face must have been flashing quickly between white pallor and red rage like a psychotic octopus on LSD."

When Dr. Lomen-Hoerth asked how he was feeling, Eric wanted to scream. *Fuck you very much for giving me a death sentence, you leering quack!* Instead, he gathered himself and responded flatly, *I am volcanically angry right now. I am only thirty-six. I got married, bought a house, have my dream career. I have just obtained my life and have only had it a few years. How is this happening to me?*

He waited for Dr. Lomen-Hoerth to concede, to repeal his diagnosis and send him and Claire on their merry way. But there is no running away from ALS. All Dr. Lomen-Hoerth could do was point to a few reasons for hope: Eric was young, healthy, and active—perhaps he would decline more slowly than most.

Eric and Claire left the office with the weight of finality that only a certified doctor can provide, and with a stack of pamphlets containing little helpful information and zero comfort. They rode the elevator in silence, and when they reached their car, Claire drove them straight to the San Francisco Zoo. "There, we tried to lose the rest of the day returning the stares of the animals in their fake environments," Eric wrote. "The animals had no comprehension or care about the anguish of two particular hairless slender humans who came to visit, so perhaps we could, for a few more hours, also have the same lack of comprehension or care. I really hoped so."

Rob Tison, diagnosed March 2010 at age thirty-nine
Asheville, North Carolina

Rob Tison left home in Commerce Township, Michigan, at age twenty-three for a job as a design engineer at Rockwell Automation in Asheville, North Carolina. His twin sister Cassie couldn't believe it.

They had hung with different crowds in high school—he was "the smart one"; she was "the social one"—but she had never considered the possibility that they wouldn't always live within a few miles of each other. The day that Rob moved, the twins and their older brother Lynn spent more than two hours in front of their parents' home, unable to let each other go. Cassie decided she would visit Rob as often as possible, and she traveled nearly every Thanksgiving for the next twenty years to see him. The annual gathering soon grew, as Cassie and her husband had four children, and, after marrying his new coworker's daughter, Rob had a son Tyler and a daughter Sydne. Then, suddenly, the family learned that it wouldn't be long before they'd never see Rob again.

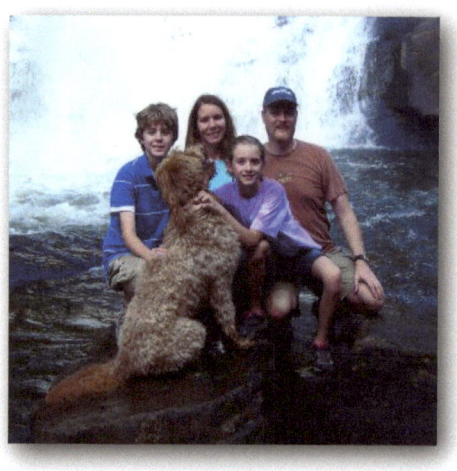

Rob Tison
With wife Kelly, kids Tyler and Sydne, and dog Otis
COURTESY OF THE TISON FAMILY

The symptoms started in late 2008. Rob began to have difficulty speaking to the point that his wife Kelly was having trouble understanding him on the phone. She'd usually blame a bad connection, and wait until he got home to talk in person. But Kelly quickly realized that the problem wasn't with their cellular service.

Doctors first diagnosed Rob's speech problems as hypothyroidism, a chemical imbalance that is fairly easy to treat with a synthetic hormone. Shortly after starting medication, however, Rob began experiencing terrible jaw spasms. When he yawned, his whole face would cramp so badly that he couldn't always keep his eyes open. Driving was an obvious risk. He switched medications, but it didn't help. Then the back of his throat started to feel strange, almost like it was sagging, he described to Kelly. That must be what was causing his difficulty speaking, he figured.

Over the next year, Rob endured a battery of exams, including a nerve conduction study and several MRIs. Despite the bizarre symptoms, all the tests came back normal. Searching for similar experiences online, he got a flood of results about bulbar-onset ALS, a form of the disease that first strikes the brain stem. In bulbar-onset ALS, motor neuron degeneration affects patients' ability to chew, swallow, and speak before spreading through the rest of the body. But there is no definitive test for ALS, and Rob's doctors weren't quite ready to levy the fatal diagnosis. "It was just kind of a wait-and-see game," Kelly recalled. "Just wait and see what the next symptom was to give us a clue as to whether he had ALS or not."

In March 2010, nearly a year and a half after his speech problems began, Rob was referred to a neurologist at Wake Forest University. Cassie flew in from Michigan and she, Rob, and Kelly traveled from Asheville to Winston-Salem to hear the final ruling: Rob had bulbar-onset ALS; he probably had less than three years to live. Cassie and Kelly sobbed. Rob, having already come to grips with his premature mortality, was stoic. At that moment, his focus was trained on his sister and wife. He wanted—needed—them to smile. As they walked back to the car, he insisted that he drive the two hours home, then let his foot rest heavy on the gas. The car accelerated as it mounted the circular ramp that climbs between levels of the parking garage, throwing the women against the side of the car and into hysterics. Rob sped around the ramp over and over again. He didn't want the laughter to stop.

BEN HARRIS, DIAGNOSED JANUARY 2011 AT AGE FORTY-FOUR
BLOOMINGTON, INDIANA

In the summer of 2010, Ben Harris found himself struggling to speak. For the first time in his life, the medical physicist had to concentrate to correctly pronounce common words as he instructed clients on how to use his company's cancer radiation equipment and software. And at a conference in Barcelona that fall, he worried that his fellow attendees would think he talked funny as he presented his oncology radiation research.

No one else seemed to notice. Ben still sounded normal; it just took more effort for him to do so. And even when his family did take note of his slowed speech, they just assumed he was carefully plotting out his answer, or coming up with something insightful to say, as he'd always done. Ben was what you might call a thinker; he had only decided to pick up a master's degree in physics, in addition to his philosophy master's, after his older brother Mike pointed out that few careers depended on training in ancient schools of thought.

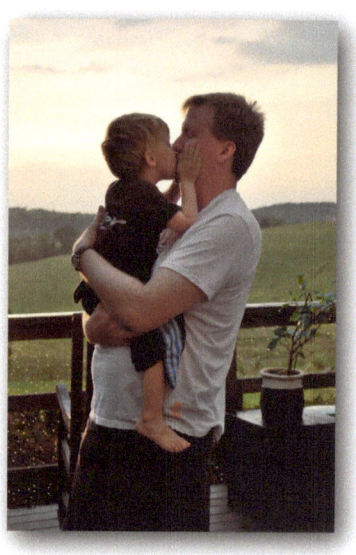

Ben Harris
With son Rawden
COURTESY OF THE
HARRIS FAMILY

But it wasn't long before the problem became more than a slight speech impairment. Ben began producing excess saliva and occasionally choking on food. Then, his tongue began visibly quivering. "I walked into the bathroom and stuck my tongue out and was horrified," he recalled. "It looked like it was full of worms." When he Googled his symptoms, he saw pages of information on bulbar-onset

Personal Trials

ALS. Reading through the results, Ben had a sinking feeling: it was a perfect match.

He raised the possibility of ALS with his wife Beccy in late December. When he showed her his tongue, she could see it wriggling, but she was reluctant to draw such a tragic conclusion. How could this wretched disease have struck so close to home? Ben didn't have a family history of the disease, but no one knows what causes ALS. Was Ben carrying a gene that increased the risk that their son Rawden, then five years old, would also develop the disease?

Ben contacted a doctor friend, who got him an appointment with a neurologist. One look at the specialist's face and Ben knew his self-diagnosis had been correct. To rule out brain cancer, the doctor ordered an MRI, which was done the same day. Both Ben and Beccy, who worked as a physician's assistant, reviewed the results themselves; their hearts sank when they didn't see a tumor. Beccy could no longer deny that her husband was in the early stages of a slow and torturous neurological decline. The next day at lunch, the couple went back to the neurologist's office for the official prognosis: rapid loss of musculature and death within three years.

"I remember I wanted to kick the wall in," said Beccy, choosing her words carefully as she relived the day that changed both their lives. "You can't make a scene, you know; that's childish."

As they came out of the doctor's office, they followed the instructions to stop at the nurses' station for the obligatory paperwork. To the people behind the desk, it was a regular day in neurology; they couldn't understand what the couple had just been through or was about to endure. "I felt we were now in very different worlds," Beccy said.

That afternoon was quiet. Ben and Beccy made phone calls to family. Beccy was still trying to wrap her mind around the situation. She had just been joking with Ben about how good things were. They'd recently moved to Bloomington, Indiana, after Ben was recruited by a new employer. They'd bought a modern split-level house, with a nice yard complete with a single-rope disc swing that Rawden loved. *They were so lucky; life couldn't be any more perfect,* Beccy remembered thinking shortly before Ben's diagnosis. "A few times I said to myself, when is something bad going to happen? When is that shoe going to drop?" she recalled. "There it was."

THIS IS THE STORY OF THREE MEN who, before the age of forty-five, received an unimaginable diagnosis. ALS is fatal. There is no cure. Most patients don't live five years after receiving a diagnosis unless they accept the necessary medical equipment to help them eat and breathe. There is only one treatment approved by the US Food and Drug Administration (FDA): riluzole, which extends the life span of ALS patients by an average of only three months. Eventually all patients must face paralysis or death. But while the disease destroys almost every last muscle in the body, it leaves the mind alert to ponder its biological imprisonment.

Eric Valor, Ben Harris, and Rob Tison refused to die without a fight—not just for their own lives, but for a disease community that for years has struggled to be heard. These three men, along with dozens of other patients suffering from ALS, researched the disease and treatments in development. And when they couldn't get their hands on an experimental drug they believed could slow their decline, they figured out what it was made of and dosed themselves with chemical substitutes purchased online.

Some called it an act of desperation. Most doctors cringed at the notion of patients self-treating with mixtures of unknown purity. But the patients supported their decisions with scientific papers and patents, and calculated their doses based on drugs in the published literature and those in clinical trials. All the while, the men tracked their results openly online, hoping their data would enlighten others and advance ALS research. Maybe their do-it-yourself approach would work, and their experiments would expedite FDA approval of an effective drug. Or maybe the treatments wouldn't help at all, and the patients' data would halt the development of a therapy that was doomed to fail. Either way, they believed the most important thing was that their efforts be shared openly with the world.

One

Clinical Optimism

Ben Harris approached the news that he had a fatal disease like he approached most things in life: with a critical eye and no-nonsense pragmatism. There wasn't much of a choice; living and dying with ALS was something he was going to have to do, and he took the assignment head-on. In early 2011, as soon as his diagnosis was official, Ben began a daily regimen of riluzole, the only approved ALS drug on the market. He also joined a site called PatientsLikeMe, which offered a platform for patients to track their health data and compare it to others'. Thousands of ALS patients had contributed data to the site, allowing the platform to display a color-coded graph of an individual's progression, relative to everyone else's.

Ben chose the screen name HappyPhysicist. It was a succinct and honest way to describe himself. He completed his profile and immediately began recording his ALS functional rating scale (FRS) score, the catch-all measure of ALS progression. It's based on a questionnaire about one's symptoms, from speech clarity to limb strength. Ben backdated an entry for the previous June, when he'd first noticed problems speaking. According to the FRS survey, he would have had the highest possible score of 48. A little icon of a man showed a green head, green torso, and green legs—Ben's whole body had been in good shape. He then completed the survey based on his current condition and added the score of 45 to his profile, dated February 4, 2011. The icon's head had changed to yellow, denoting the trouble Ben had been having with his speech and ability to swallow.

According to the automatically generated chart, his rate of progression put him on par with the 75th percentile of ALS patients on the site: his body was declining a little more slowly than most, but he was still within the average range. For his status, he selected "feeling good." "I can still work and play with my son," he wrote. But the chart also projected his future decline, and the outlook was dismal. In less than three years, his FRS score would bottom out, and he wasn't likely to live to see it reach zero.

He and his wife Beccy started attending support groups, but she found them depressing. She saw their future in the other patients and spouses, and felt the blow of the diagnosis all over again. She wanted to be there for Ben, but she always ended up feeling worse after the group discussions. Ben saw her pain and convinced her to let him go alone. Eventually, he stopped attending too.

Instead, Ben found support online. In addition to tracking his data, he joined an active community of ALS patients on forums hosted by PatientsLikeMe and other sites. The discussion boards not only offered advice on dealing with ALS, but also provided information about the disease and possible remedies. In-depth exchanges about alternative and experimental treatments for ALS augmented Ben's own research and led him to a number of promising options. Ben experimented with various supplements, including vitamin C, melatonin, and a compound meant to boost the health of the mitochondria, the energy-producing organelles of the cell. "At first I just tried anything that I could find a theoretical argument for," Ben said. Despite these efforts, however, his condition continued to decline. By March, he was losing strength in his left arm and leg, and his FRS score had dropped another point.

He decided to enroll in a clinical study for an experimental new drug for ALS. He knew of two trials recruiting ALS patients, and he was eligible for both. Palo Alto–based Neuraltus Pharmaceuticals was testing an infusion therapy called NP001. It had yielded positive results in a Phase 1 safety trial and slowed the disease in mice, most likely by reducing neurotoxic inflammation. The Phase 2 trial would deliver six rounds of infusions over as many months, and the University of Kentucky in Lexington, just a three-hour drive from Ben's home in Bloomington, Indiana, was a participating center.

Meanwhile, Knopp Biosciences and Biogen Idec were looking for ALS patients to take part in their Phase 3 trial for dexpramipexole (dex), an oral therapy believed to improve mitochondrial health and ward off neuron death. Phase 2 trial participants receiving the higher dose had slowed decline and longer survival.[1] The Washington University School of Medicine in St. Louis, one of the centers hosting the Phase 3, was less than four hours from Bloomington. Undecided, Ben screened for both trials.

After doing hours of research and reading dozens of patient testimonials online, Ben settled on joining the dex trial. Both new drugs seemed promising, but dex was further along in development, which meant there was already some evidence suggesting that it worked in humans. The trial's later stage also meant that, if all went well, the drug was closer to FDA approval. NP001, on the other hand, was still years from hitting the market, so there was a chance he wouldn't be able to continue taking the drug after the trial was over, even if it helped stem his disease. Then, on the night of June 9, Ben got a galvanizing email from Rob Tison, an ALS patient in North Carolina who had recently begun his infusions as part of the ongoing NP001 trial: the drug was working.

Rob was about the same age as Ben, also had bulbar-onset ALS, and, according to his charts on PatientsLikeMe, had a similar rate of progression. Rob had received his first infusion of NP001 just three days earlier, and already he was experiencing dramatic improvements. In his email to Ben, he emphasized his much-improved ability to swallow. It had been at least six months, probably a year, since he'd been able to drink fluids normally, he said; he was forced to slurp and gulp, and he never managed more than about a half cup a minute. "I can only take in small sips as my muscles try to 'fight' me," Rob wrote. But on the morning of his third infusion, all that had changed. "Multiple times during the day yesterday, and still today, I am surprised to drink liquids normally. I know it sounds crazy and unbelievable, but it is true."

Rob also spoke of a "more productive" cough and "greater strength and dexterity" in his right arm and hand. He could once again use his right hand to shift gears while driving to and from the hospital, and dressing himself that morning had been shockingly easy. NP001 wasn't just slowing his progression, it was actually reversing it—something no ALS drug had ever done. "Again, I realize this sounds too good to be true, and I would flat-out think it impossible if I were not in my body."

Ben promptly forgot why he'd decided on the dexpramipexole trial. One week later, he signed up for a chance to try NP001 for himself. He received his first infusion the following Monday.

Two

Learning to live with ALS

In 2005, six years before Ben joined the NP001 trial, Eric took his ALS diagnosis with a similar can-do spirit. He wanted to know everything there was to know about the disease—what initiated it; how it manifested at a cellular level; what it would do to his body, and when. He scheduled his regular checkups with the head nurse at the University of California, San Francisco clinic for the last appointment of the day, so he could "mercilessly pick her brain while she closed the office." He was intelligent and charming, and she helped as best she could. Unfortunately, most of his questions couldn't be answered.

He started taking riluzole immediately and joined a trial for an experimental drug called ritonavir. Eric was put into the high-dose group, receiving 400 milligrams of ritonavir twice daily for six months. Of course, he didn't know it at the time because, like many clinical trials, this one was blinded. Neither Eric nor his doctor were told which dose he was getting—high, low, or placebo—until after the data had been analyzed. Had Eric known at the beginning of the trial that he was getting the drug, he would have been pleased; trial participants understandably prefer to try the new therapy that may help them, rather than a sugar pill that merely serves as a statistical control in the name of science. However, after an interim safety analysis the researchers found that the drug had failed to help. In fact, the higher dose had accelerated disease progression. Patients in that group averaged a five-fold greater decline in lung capacity, a nineteen-fold greater decline in weight, and a three-fold greater decline in strength compared with the placebo group.[2] The trial was terminated early, but as one of the first patients enrolled, Eric had already completed a full course of the drug.

Undeterred, Eric enrolled in another study, one for a natural antioxidant called Coenzyme Q10. He was again randomly selected to get the treatment rather than a placebo; this time, the treatment was shown to be ineffective.[3] Indeed, nothing seemed to work. Eric's left foot continued to drag, and his right foot followed suit. His arms and hands grew weaker, and his speech started to slur. For a while, he was able to hide his symptoms. But as his right thigh began to deteriorate, he was forced to support his weight with a cane. "I remember getting funny looks doing Christmas shopping at Stanford Mall, a high end shopping center," he said. "An otherwise athletic thirty-seven-year-old man in fashionable business casual with a cane was obviously an affectation, right?"

As the muscles of his tongue and jaw wasted away, it became progressively harder for him to eat. Once an avid surfer, snowboarder, and skateboarder, he had been a well-built 170 or 180 pounds. But by 2006, the weight began melting off. After losing 25 pounds in less than two months, he scheduled surgery to have a feeding tube implanted so he could supplement what he ate with liquids pumped directly into his stomach. The following year, his declining leg strength forced him to use a walker or crutches, which challenged his navigation on the numerous stairs in his prized Santa Cruz beach cottage. He could

Personal Trials

make it up and down short flights by leaning on the banister, but that wouldn't last. He and his wife Claire would have to move. And to afford another residence in Northern California, they'd have to sell.

It pained Eric to part with the house he'd spent so many hours working on, and to move away from the beach to which he and Claire had so often escaped with their surfboards. But they were lucky to find a ranch-style house only a mile down the road that the owner sold to them for nearly $100,000 less than market value, Eric said, largely out of sympathy for his condition. His stepdad Floyd remodeled the bathroom, and the rest of the house was already wheelchair accessible. It would only be another few months until Eric was unable to stand.

Just seven months before receiving his diagnosis, Eric had landed a job as the senior systems administrator of research and development at DaimlerChrysler, maker of Mercedes Benz before the two automotive giants split in May 2007. The work involved managing all of the office's computers, networks, and telephones, and improving communication between the Palo Alto, Sacramento, Portland, and Long Beach branches. He also helped set up the computer systems that led to innovations such as Google Maps integration and automatic safety systems like collision avoidance. "That job was my ultimate joy," he said—"cars and computers and German beer."

But his career was next on ALS's path of destruction. By late 2007, Eric could no longer hold the steering wheel of his car; he had to be dropped off each morning by Claire or his mother on the way to their respective workplaces. A coworker would meet Eric outside with the power wheelchair he kept in his office and help get him from the car to the chair. The company accommodated Eric's growing disability, allowing him to move offices twice. But his situation was unsustainable. When Eric finally retired in February 2008, he was using a chopstick to type.

Soon thereafter, Eric was forced to take the next major step in his ALS journey: a tracheotomy. He scheduled the procedure after a blockage in his airway nearly took his life. "It's much better than an emergency situation," he said.

As his arms grew too weak to manipulate a mouse, he learned to navigate his computer using an eye-gaze camera called ERICA, which directed the cursor by tracking the movement of his right eye and provided an on-screen keyboard for

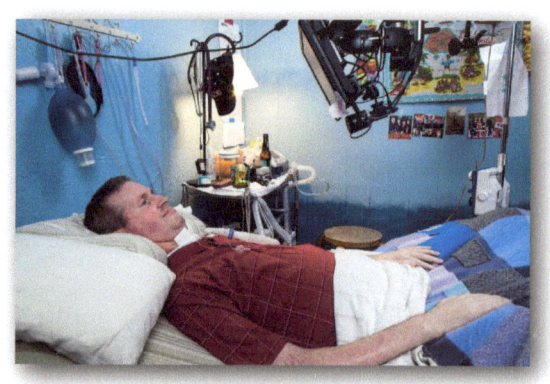

In his home, February 2013
© ELIOT DRAKE

him to type. The technology also gave him a voice by allowing him to write out his thoughts for the computer to read aloud to others in the room or to people on the phone.

Bedridden and jobless, Eric dove headfirst into his ALS research. He scoured PubMed, a database of peer-reviewed scientific articles, for clues about what causes ALS and how to stop the decline. He'd save dozens of manuscripts to his desktop, later combing them for new information about the disease. When he found something of interest, he'd write to the scientists with questions about their research. He shared what he learned with other patients online, and in 2009 he started a blog to publish his work. And whenever he found a treatment that he thought would be worth trying, he'd try it. For him, there was no conflict in playing both researcher and patient. "As some people can attest, I have an ability to be a cold bastard," he said. "I just treat myself as another lab rat."

As if battling a life-threatening disease wasn't enough of a burden on his family, Eric's physical decline continued to translate into significant financial troubles. He soon required full-time in-home care, which was not covered by insurance. By 2010, he and Claire had eaten through their savings and were forced to sell their house yet again, just to afford another six or eight months of care. Unfortunately, "the week that we put our house on the market, two other houses in our immediate area went into foreclosure and the prices plummeted," Eric said. "We ended up having to short-sell, which eliminated all of the equity—and our caretaker money." He made arrangements for them to move in with his mom Joan and stepdad Floyd in a house just outside of town that had a separate apartment. Floyd once again remodeled the bathroom for Eric, and the family moved the day before Thanksgiving 2010. That's when things took a turn for the worse.

Eric became less and less responsive over the course of the weekend. Claire brought a urine sample for testing, and Joan received a call from the doctor as soon as the results were in. *His blood sugar is really high,* he told her. *I think his kidneys are shutting down, and he may be leaving us.* Joan rushed Eric to the hospital, where she was told that his body was failing. The doctors didn't expect him to last the night.

But he did. By morning, his blood sugar had dropped and his liver function had rebounded. After three days in the hospital, Eric was prescribed insulin and diabetes medication to control his glucose levels, and was finally allowed to go to his new home. It would feel empty when he got there, though: Claire was gone. Between the loss of their house and watching Eric's decline, the situation had become too much for her.

After the dust settled, and Eric, Joan, and Floyd got accustomed to life in their new environment, one ray of hope remained. That summer, Eric had stumbled across Neuraltus's NP001. The company claimed that it targeted the body's macrophages, immune cells most commonly known for engulfing and digesting cellular debris and pathogens. One theory of ALS was that an overly zealous inflammatory reaction was triggering the neurodegeneration that causes paralysis, and that macrophages were to blame. The cells were stuck in an activated state that somehow damages motor neurons, researchers said. Experiments suggested that NP001 flipped a switch in macrophages so that instead of causing inflammation they helped reduce it by gobbling up pathogens, dead cells, and toxins.

On June 16, 2011, Eric used the eye-gaze technology mounted above his bed to start a new forum discussion on the website of the ALS Therapy Development Institute (ALS TDI): "Has anyone heard of Neuraltus or their product NP001?" he asked. "Searches for those terms turned up nothing here."

An hour later, another forum user shared a link to the trial's description on clinicaltrials.gov, a nationwide registry run by the National Library of Medicine.[4] Others soon weighed in. Some patients reached out to the company for more information and received

Personal Trials

confirmation that a Phase 1 safety trial was imminent; a larger Phase 2 study was expected soon after. The forum buzzed with questions, skepticism, frustration, and excitement. Targeting the immune system to slow or stop ALS progression was a relatively new idea, but already there were multiple immune-modulating therapies being explored. And Neuraltus, at least, had secured $17 million to fund the development of NP001.

Unfortunately, Eric—ventilated and confined to his bed—was far too advanced in his disease to qualify as a trial participant. His speech was barely intelligible, and he was unable to move any part of his body except for his eyes and some of the muscles of his face. "I am considered 'dead' for the purposes of clinical trials," he said. But maybe there was another option.

While the company had not disclosed the details of NP001's composition, Eric and his fellow forum contributors scoured the scientific literature for more information. In early August, the group uncovered a handful of studies by Neuraltus cofounder Michael McGrath on a chlorite-based drug called WF10. It had been developed in the late 1990s by a company called Oxo Chemie, where Dr. McGrath had been the chief scientific officer, and it had already been approved in Thailand for treating the autoimmune consequences of cancer radiation. WF10 had also been tested extensively for its utility in treating HIV, but had failed to show efficacy in a Phase 3 trial in 2004.

Eric wondered if NP001 might be some sort of WF10 derivative. Maybe NP001 also contained chlorite in some form. More importantly, if both NP001 and WF10 were chlorite-based, and if NP001 turned out to successfully treat ALS, could WF10 prove just as good?

Photos courtesy of the Valor family

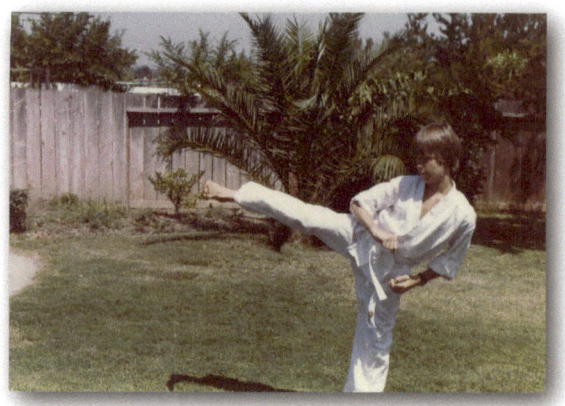

Summer 1980

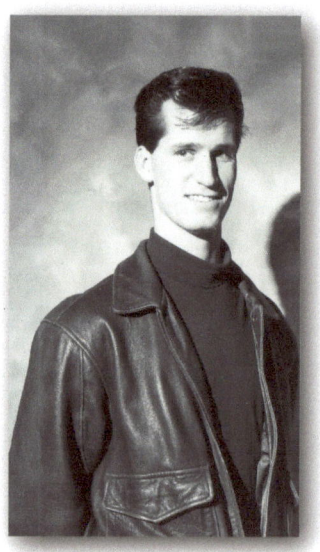

1990

Personal Trials

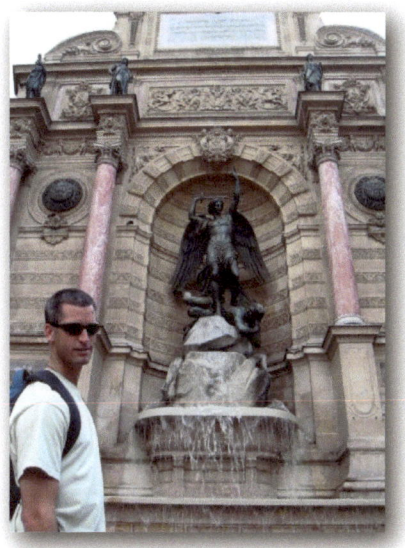

Paris, France, 2002

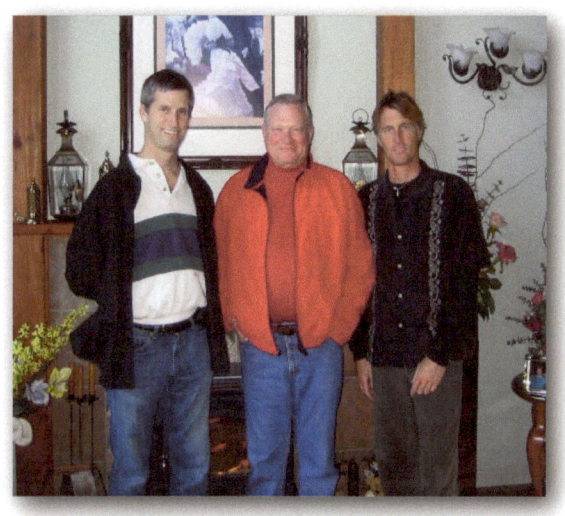

With dad Norm and brother Scott, early 2005

Jef Akst

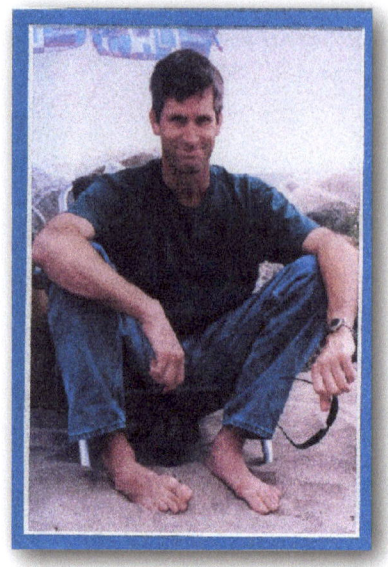

At the beach shortly after diagnosis, summer 2005

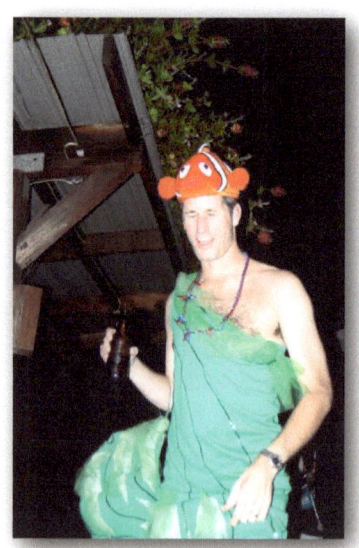

Halloween 2005

Personal Trials

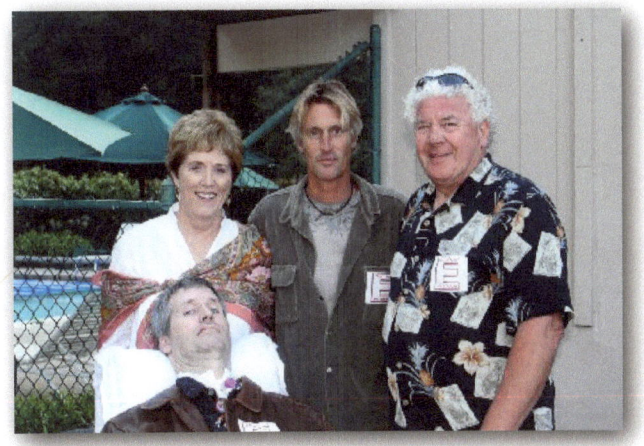

With mom Joan, brother Scott, and stepdad Floyd, at a fundraiser on his 40th birthday, fall 2008

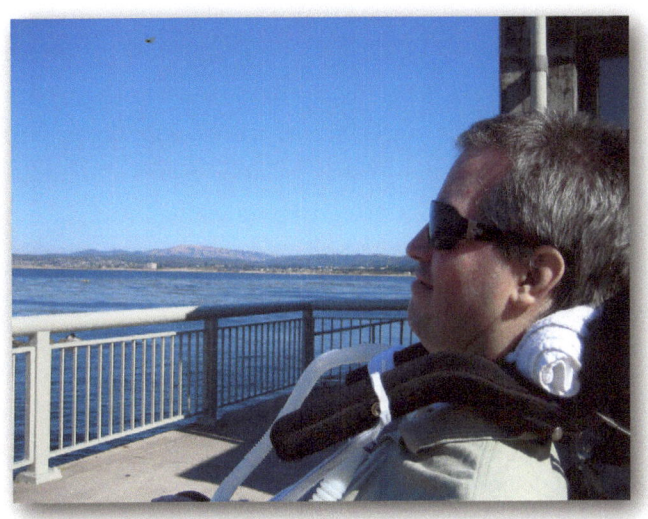

Spring 2012

Three

Hidden treasure?

By early September 2010, Neuraltus had treated most of the thirty-two participants in its Phase 1 trial. Each patient received a single infusion of NP001 in one of four doses. Many patients involved in the trial posted progress reports on the forums; Eric also relayed updates he received personally. By all accounts, no serious adverse events occurred that would stop the company from moving the drug forward into a Phase 2 trial, which would involve more patients and more infusions of NP001 for each.

Meanwhile, Eric and other forum contributors, including Rob Tison (known online as Persevering), continued to share whatever information they could find on the drug and its maker. Evidence mounted that NP001 was a chlorite-based solution, perhaps a refined version of WF10. Especially convincing was a copy of a trial consent form that seemingly made the claim that NP001 was, simply, sodium chlorite: "The purpose of this study is to test NP001 (sodium chlorite) to determine if it is safe and tolerable in patients with ALS."

Personal Trials

In October, Neuraltus presented an update on its neurodegenerative disease drug pipeline, including NP001, at the BIO Investor Forum in San Francisco. Eager to see if the company had mentioned the results of the Phase 1 trial, Rob got hold of the presentation. Sure enough, the slides did mention the recent study, and the results looked promising. But immediately, Rob noted something a bit off. One graph depicted a patient's decline, then a dramatic plateau during a seven-month treatment period, followed by seven months of observation. The Phase 1 trial had only begun that year—too recently for the company to be reporting fourteen months' worth of data. Moreover, the graph depicted five treatments, whereas the Phase 1 trial protocol stated that patients would receive only a single dose. "Seems odd that they just completed Phase 1 and their data doesn't fit the protocol," Rob wrote on the forum.

He wondered if perhaps the data didn't come from the recent trial. The graph was titled "Experience of an ALS Patient Treated with NP001 Active Moiety," whatever that was. But the slides just before and after the graph did refer to the Phase 1 study, so Rob was unsure. He emailed the presentation to Eric, who also noted the discrepancy. He speculated that perhaps the first four treatments were actually WF10 or another chlorite drug, and only the last dose was NP001, but that didn't make much sense either.

On November 30, the company formally announced its Phase 1 trial results, which confirmed that patients had only received a single dose of NP001. The study found the drug to be safe at all four doses tested, and revealed a dose-dependent change in a suspected ALS biomarker—a promising sign that the drug might slow ALS progression. But there was no reference to patients that had tried longer treatment courses of NP001 or WF10. The results that Neuraltus had presented the month before were not mentioned at all.

The next day the patients got their answer. Rob found a patent granted to Neuraltus cofounder Michael McGrath entitled "Chlorite in the treatment of neurodegenerative disease."[5] The patent application, filed back in January 2005, included what appeared to be the very same data depicted in the October presentation, but it contained much more information. The patient hadn't been treated with NP001 at all—it didn't exist then; the entire treatment course had been with WF10. According to the patent, the patient was a fifty-nine-year-old woman with a familial form of ALS. In less than two years, she had declined from an FRS of 40 (the highest score on the version of the scale used at the time) to just 15. She could no longer swallow foods or fluids and was surviving on a feeding tube. But after five infusions of WF10, she regained the ability to eat, and her feeding tube was removed. Her facial muscles stopped twitching, and her voice grew steadier. She completed four more cycles of WF10. During the therapy and for about two months after, her FRS score did not decline at all. A few months after her fifth and last treatment of WF10, however, she began to regress at a rate identical to her pretreatment progression. She died six months later. The discontinuation of treatment was simply attributed to the patient's inability to obtain the drug.

Rob compared the data on the woman's progression from the patent to the data on the slide from Neuraltus's presentation. He could see that they were a match, offset by ten and a half months, and with a few minor deviations, which he attributed to the poor image quality of the graphs. He was convinced the patients were one and the same. Neuraltus had chosen to share data on someone taking WF10 in a presentation about NP001, supporting his long-held suspicions that NP001 was indeed a chlorite-based drug. Another relevant patent noted the high pH of WF10, and the pain this caused some patients at the infusion site, leading Rob to suggest that NP001 might be a more neutral version of the drug.[6] "It seems that NP001 is essentially

WF10 that is a higher purity of the good stuff, without the small portion of bad 'contaminants' and perhaps with a buffer for pH level," he wrote to the group.

More importantly, the dramatic improvement that WF10 apparently provided some ALS patients reinforced Eric's original hope that this older drug, which was available for purchase in Thailand, might stall ALS progression. In addition to the fifty-nine-year-old female patient, the patent described the improvement of a thirty-seven-year-old man who was diagnosed with ALS in 2003. The disease progressed rapidly until he began a regimen of WF10 a year later. Within a week, he regained his ability to eat, his feeding tube was removed, and he remained stable at a point in his disease where he could still walk with a walker, the patent stated. And in a *San Francisco Business Times* article published shortly after the October presentation,[7] then Neuraltus CEO Andrew Gengos alluded to a third patient who experienced spontaneous remission after taking WF10.

"It is amazing that a drug with this potential, as evidenced in the patent data from more than six years ago, and on the shelf was 'hidden,' " Rob wrote on the forum. "If this is REAL, this is amazing as well as amazingly frustrating that this data is older than the patent application of 2005. There may already be a very effective treatment that is commercially available."

———

A couple of weeks later, Rob attended the Motor Neuron Disease Association's International Symposium in Orlando, where he tracked down Michael McGrath and Ari Azhir, two Neuraltus cofounders who were presenting a poster on NP001. He wanted to pick their brains about the drug and the company's plans for its development. He had a noticeable limp, but was still quick on his feet. His smile projected a youthful spirit, but the strawberry blond male-pattern baldness on his head divulged his true age. He eagerly approached them, iPad in hand. His speech was so belabored by this time that he preferred to type his conversations.

He impressed the researchers with his extensive knowledge of immune-modulating treatments for ALS, and about NP001 specifically. Few patients interested in an experimental drug had read all of the patents underlying its development. Rob was similarly impressed by McGrath and Azhir, who seemed committed to NP001's success. He was particularly excited to learn that the researchers knew of the forum's discussions. ("They were aware of this thread!" he posted that night.) But most rewarding were the details they provided him about NP001. "Dr. McGrath confirmed that NP001 is a pure chlorite with a more neutral pH to avoid burns at the IV site, as compared to WF10," Rob wrote. "So, the assumptions of the related patents were spot on."

Rob learned that the company planned to begin a Phase 2 study the following year at about twenty locations. It would include 120 patients, a third of whom would receive a placebo. Unfortunately, he also learned that patients more than two years removed from their first symptoms would be ineligible, as was common in ALS drug trials. By the time the study was expected to start, it would have been at least that long since Rob had first begun to feel "off"; he didn't think he would be accepted. And he knew that many patients on the forums would also be excluded for being too advanced in their disease.

His next question, then, was whether the company would consider an expanded access program, sometimes called compassionate use, allowing patients not involved in the trial to receive the drug. Many biomedical companies don't like to grant access to their experimental drugs before market approval; more people using a drug increases the chances of an adverse effect, which could cause unwanted delays or even derail a clinical program. With hundreds of millions or billions of dollars invested, companies understandably want to reduce those risks until they can recoup their investment. And although the FDA allows companies to charge for the cost of manufacturing drugs made available through an expanded access program, for a small biotech company focused on making enough to complete another clinical trial, ancillary expenses can be prohibitive.

But the Neuraltus cofounders told Rob that they hoped expanded access would be available following the Phase 2 trial. "Dr. Azhir is a very caring lady, genuinely concerned about helping ALS patients," Rob told the forum. "She is already planning to pursue whatever is necessary to enable the compassionate use of NP001 following Phase 2."

But having not even begun, the trial wouldn't be complete for at least a year, probably closer to two. WF10 was available now. Patients began researching how they might be able to get the older chlorite drug for themselves. On the evening of January 23, a forum contributor from Spain posted what seemed to be good news—an email he had received from a Thai company called Biomaxx that claimed to have used the drug to successfully treat ALS. The lengthy note, written in imperfect English, read like something out of a marketing campaign:

> Yes we use Immunokine (WF10) more than 10 years and we have very good experience with this preparation by different types of cancer, by chronic inflammations and also by chronic infections but only by round about 40 ALS patients within the last 3 years. That's not a lot of patients but we can say in general Immunokine is very helpful and can reduce or eliminate the symptoms. That means one of the most important results is a better life quality and in conclusion our data show that under the conditions used it may inhibit the expected effects.

Inhibit disease progression? Reduce or eliminate the symptoms? It sounded too good to be true, and most on the forum suspected that it was. But if it really was WF10, at least this guy was willing to sell it: "The patient can do everything in home situation," the email continued, "just an educated nurse should setup the infusion; intravenously but absolute harmless."

Of course, there was the matter of payment. In a section of the email fittingly mislabeled "Expensive," rather than "Expense," the email outlined the calculations, and determined that for a patient weighing approximately 50 kilograms (110 pounds), the WF10 treatment—along with the accompanying doses of vitamins C, B1, B6, and B12, and glutathione that the company recommended—would cost €13,530. Shipping to Europe would be an additional €250. Eric quickly did the math: it was around $19,000. Payment was required in advance.

Some on the forum wondered if the drug actually cost that much, or if the company had marked it up to make some extra money. Other patients who had reached out to Biomaxx were getting similar emails, signed by someone named Dr. Trogisch, but with different prices and sometimes different dosage protocols. Rob noted the discrepancies and warned the group to proceed with caution. "Without any stated valid reason, he has more frequent and greater dosing than has ever been mentioned in the numerous clinical studies conducted for other ailments or related patent documents," Rob wrote. "I am not a doctor, but if I were to try it, I'd be careful to avoid his 'extras' and stick with the dose amount and frequency quoted so many times."

A couple of days later, a forum contributor named Bubba received an email that validated the patients' concerns. It was from Dr. Friedrich-Wilhelm Kuehne, the inventor of WF10; he still used the drug to treat autoimmune diseases and cancer as part of his company OXO Chemie, also located in Thailand:

Today (25.1.2011) it came to my attention that a Mr. Trogisch from Bangkok claims to have used a drug named Immunokine (codename WF10) for the treatment of 40 patients suffering from amyotrophic lateral sclerosis (ALS) during the last 3 years. I am the inventor and developer of this drug WF10 for more than 30 years. And I consider it my duty to inform you that Mr. Trogisch's claims are untrue. He has not treated one single ALS diagnosed patient.

Dr. Kuehne confirmed that only a few ALS patients had ever been treated with WF10, and that their data had been included in the patent filed by Neuraltus cofounder Michael McGrath. The patients had reported "a tingling sensation in the extremities" as well as "increasing strength already after the first infusion cycle," he said. While it was illegal to ship to the United States, he could provide WF10 on an off-label basis to patients in Europe and Thailand.

The very same week that the emails from Biomaxx and OXO Chemie circulated on the forum, Neuraltus announced that it would begin recruiting patients for a Phase 2 trial.

Rob was devastated that he was not eligible for the new NP001 study. And angry. It didn't seem fair for yet another card to be stacked against him—and all ALS victims. It often takes more than a year to diagnose the disease, leaving patients with less than a year of trial eligibility. Rob was only ten months removed from his diagnosis, yet according to the trial rules, he was already ineligible.

After hearing Dr. Richard "Rick" Bedlack of the Duke ALS Clinic give a talk about low enrollment in ALS trials, Rob decided to air his grievances. He reached out to Dr. Bedlack to see if there was any way to "reverse this terrible trend that is ridiculously limiting clinical study eligibility." In addition to being exceedingly frustrating to ALS patients desperate to try new therapies, the strict inclusion criteria may cherry-pick patients who progress unusually fast and tend to get a quicker diagnosis, leaving a longer window of trial eligibility, Rob noted. If fast progressors are less likely to respond a drug, "this may even bias their results toward failure," he added.

That May, while attending National ALS Advocacy Day in Washington, DC, Dr. Bedlack found Rob and his wife Kelly eating lunch on the lawn. By this time, Rob had severely limited mobility. He was still able to walk with the support of a cane, but he had also purchased an electric wheelchair. He had hesitated to take it into the city that day, but fortunately his family had insisted. Rob scooted many miles around the streets of the nation's capital, a satisfied grin plastered across his face.

He was in good spirits when Dr. Bedlack pulled up a seat next to him. They talked for more than an hour. Over the course of their conversation and an email exchange that followed, Dr. Bedlack realized that Rob was counting his first symptoms

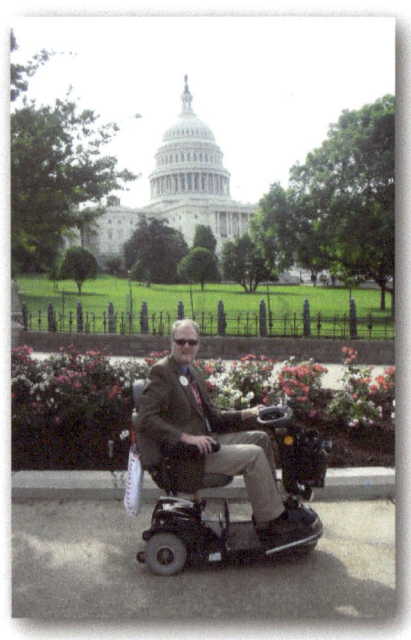

At ALS Association Advocacy weekend in Washington, DC, May 2011
COURTESY OF THE TISON FAMILY

as any "funny feeling" that, in retrospect, may have been very early signs of ALS. But in the context of clinical trials, Dr. Bedlack said, it's really the first unexplained weakness that defines disease onset. By this standard, he reasoned, Rob still qualified for the Phase 2 trial.

Rob was elated. He immediately made arrangements to visit the Duke clinic, where the study coordinator took his vitals and reviewed the consent forms with him. She answered his many questions about the drug and ran him through a series of tests to confirm his eligibility for the trial. He returned less than two weeks later for the NP001 treatment that would send signs of life shooting through his body.

Photos courtesy of the Tison family

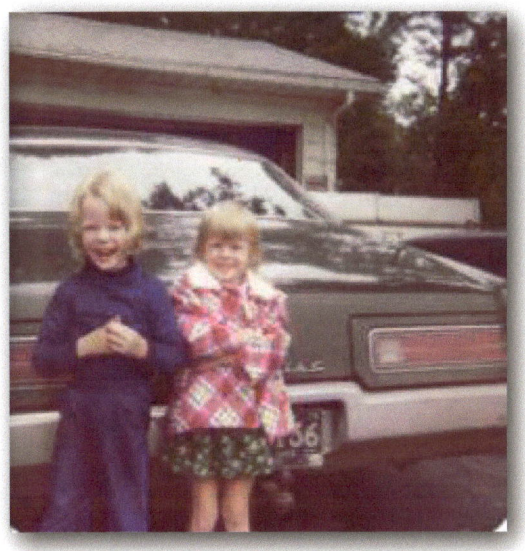

With twin sister Cassie in front of
their family home in Commerce
Township, Michigan, circa 1973

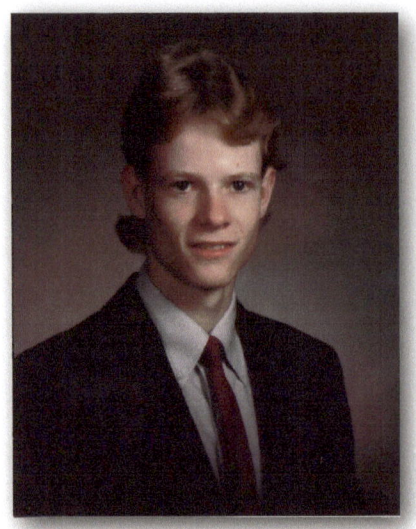

As a high school senior, 1987-1988

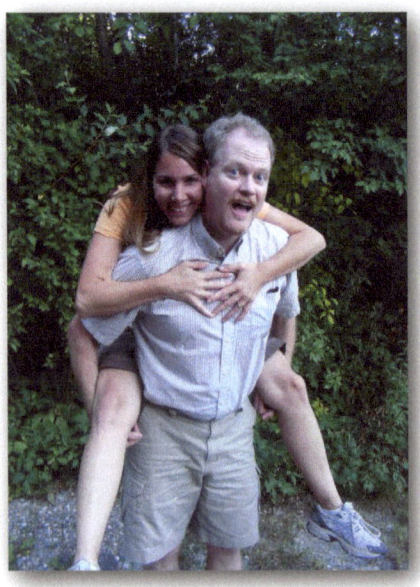

Proving that he was still strong enough to pick up wife Kelly, August 2010

Personal Trials

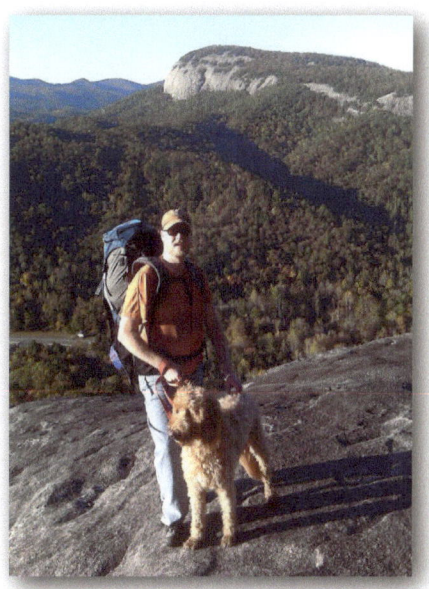

Backpacking in the Appalachian Mountains of western North Carolina, October 2010

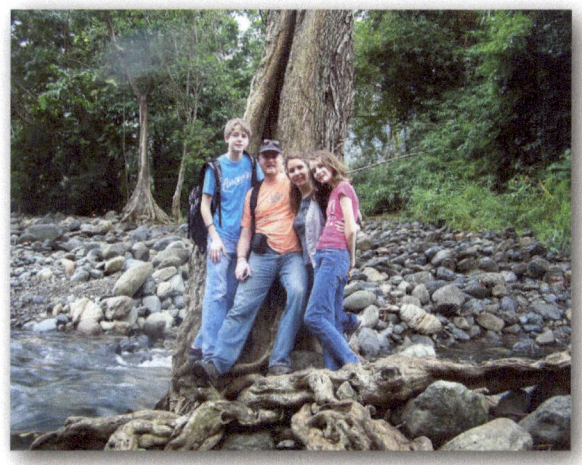

On vacation with wife Kelly and kids Tyler and Sydne in Puerto Rico, December 2010

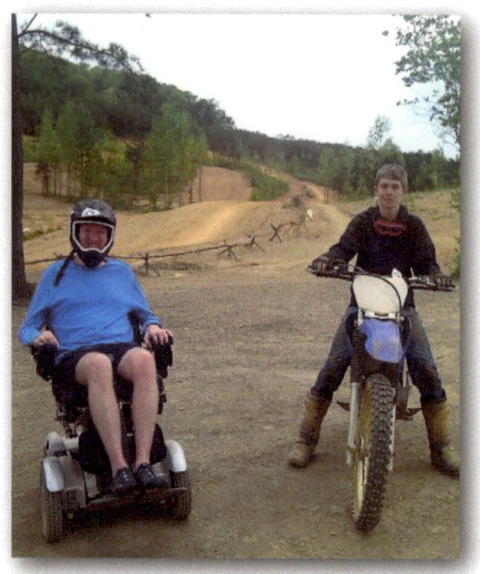

With son Tyler, April 2012

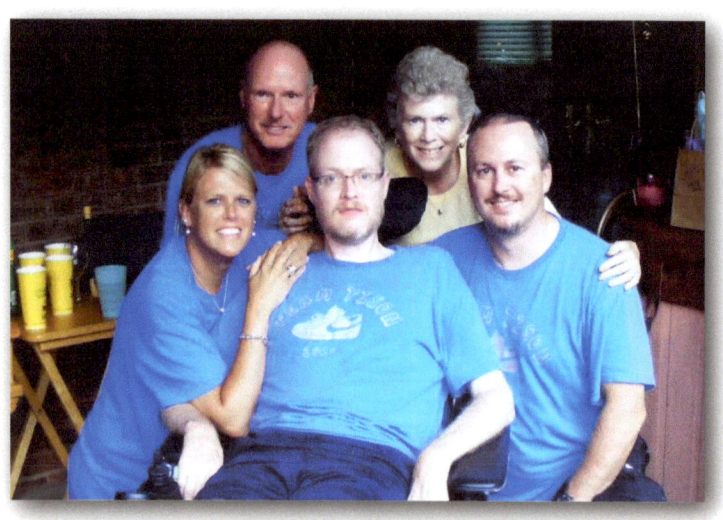

With parents, twin sister Cassie, and big brother Lynn on Rob and Cassie's 42nd birthday, June 2012

Personal Trials

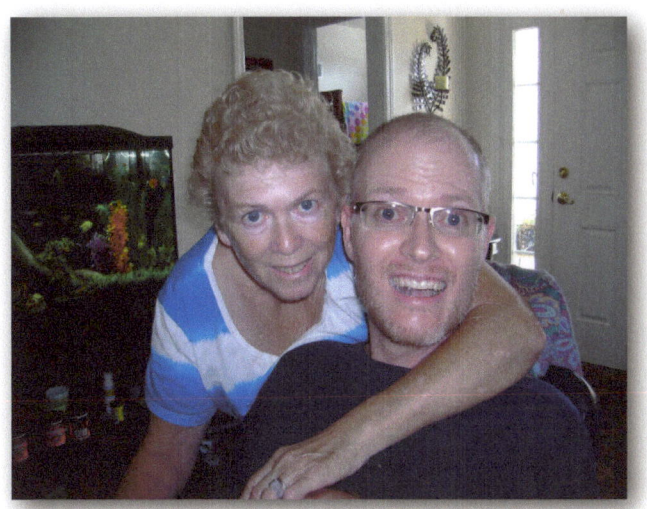

With mom Barbara, August 2012

Four

An infusion of hope

On June 19, 2011, Ben drove three hours through the midwestern countryside to Lexington, Kentucky. His first trial treatment was scheduled for the next morning, so he checked in at his hotel and tried to get a little rest. When the time came, he headed to the University of Kentucky health care center. He wore a neatly pressed button-down shirt; his short red hair was slicked to one side. He surveyed the sprawling red brick complex from the grass across from the main entrance and snapped a few photos for posterity. Then he headed inside for his first infusion of NP001.

He checked in at the front desk and followed a nurse down the hall to a small exam room. She motioned for him to have a seat in the green vinyl medical chair and made small talk as she set up his IV. When she was finished, she offered him something to drink, then left the room. Ben pulled out his laptop to get some work done while the medicine dripped into his bloodstream.

That afternoon and into the evening, Ben kept waiting for the fatigue to set in. Rob had told him that the infusions had made him tired,

Personal Trials

and Ben expected to experience the same side effect if he was lucky enough to receive NP001 and not the placebo. But he felt fine. "I felt as chipper as a bushy tailed bunny all night after the first infusion," he told the forum. *What a waste,* he thought. *Driving three hours each way to spend more than three weeks in a hotel room in Kentucky just to be injected with salt water.* Heading back to the clinic for his second infusion the next day was about the hardest thing he'd ever done. But it was too soon to draw any conclusions about his treatment, and even if he was getting the placebo, science must go on. He wasn't about to quit now.

After setting up his IV, the nurse again offered him a drink. He accepted; if he wasn't getting chlorite then at least he could down some caffeine. *Coffee, please,* he said, speaking slowly so that she could understand his low, muffled voice. After a moment, the nurse returned with his coffee, and Ben pulled out his laptop.

A few minutes later, Ben distractedly reached for the coffee and was shocked to find that it was empty. He had drunk the whole thing without even noticing! He did a double take, confirming that the cup was indeed void of all liquid. He couldn't believe it. "I had not been able to drink without my full concentration in about three months," Ben later told his baby brother Jason, an amateur filmmaker who was documenting Ben's decline. "If I had drunk liquid without paying attention, I would choke. It would be a dramatic, terrifying choking scene. And now I was sitting, staring at an empty cup of coffee that I drank without thinking. To me, that was impossible." Instantly, Ben knew that he was getting the drug, and that the drug was working.

After the infusion, Ben, who had joined the study coordinator for lunch, began testing himself. He tilted his head back further and took bigger gulps of water without any problems. Then he decided to really push the limit: he fixed his gaze on a ceiling tile and chugged. "It felt like jumping off a cliff," he wrote to Rob in an email that afternoon. "I was afraid I might cough it all up into the study coordinator's face but I just had to know that instant if the improvement was real. To my utter amazement I chugged the liquid easily!"

His muscle twitches had also subsided, he was drooling less, and his tongue had increased range of motion. Consuming solid foods had once "been about as easy as mud wrestling a walrus and took the concentration of a tight rope walker," he told Rob. "Now, I munched away focusing less and less on the task of eating."

He also noticed a slight improvement in his speech. When he arrived back home, he found that he could once again make the hard "T" sound in "Otis," the name of the family basset hound, and he could speak for extended periods of time without tiring. "Asking me to have a short polite conversation was like asking me to load up a pickup truck with 20-lb bags of sand. I dreaded it and it exhausted me. Even after just a couple of sentences my jaw would be sore," Ben said. "This afternoon, I couldn't stop talking. My speech is still impaired but I can talk now for much longer."

The changes were unmistakable. Just as Rob had experienced, the drug wasn't simply stalling Ben's progression, it was actually reversing it.

Ben was ecstatic as he and Beccy headed off with young Rawden to Sedona, Arizona, for a big Harris family reunion. All five of Ben's siblings were there, as were both of his parents, who had been separated for more than thirty years. It had been a decade since the family last gathered. After Ben's diagnosis, they'd all agreed to get together yearly.

Ben was the second youngest of the six kids, and growing up, the house had never been quiet. Each sibling would often have two or three friends over, making the Harris home a full-out block party.

Personal Trials

With the extended family, including spouses and ten grandkids, gathered in Sedona, the rental house took on a similar vibe. The group decided to rekindle an old beef between Ben and Jason: Who could make a better pizza? The week was dedicated to planning, executing, and tasting the cook-off. Jason, of course, filmed the whole thing. In the end, Ben reigned as champion.

When Ben shared the news of NP001's dramatic effect, the family was thrilled. Who knew what would happen in the long run, but the fact that Ben was feeling better than he had in months was cause enough for celebration. The group rented a jeep and took turns gunning the vehicle over the rocks and divots of the red-dirt trail. Later, they hiked up to the towering structures of Cathedral Rock, where they had a nearly 360-degree view of the red desert landscape. With his newfound energy, Ben powered up the steep hillside with the rest of his family. At the summit, he sat on a rock wall, his legs dangling over the edge of the canyon, and hammed it up for the camera. He repeatedly shaded his eyes with one hand or the other as he stared out at the abyss in front of him, as if he was saluting the desert itself. He looked on top of the world.

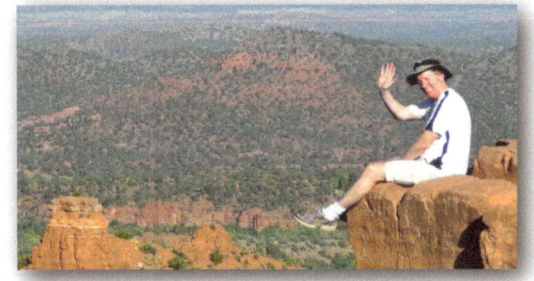
At Cathedral Rock in Sedona, Arizona, June 2011
COURTESY OF THE HARRIS FAMILY

After a couple of weeks, the effects started to fade. But Ben's next round of infusions in July delivered a similar pick-me-up.

His mouth and throat began to work properly, so that he could once again gargle without spitting all over the sink. He stopped biting his lower lip when he spoke and ate, and he could purse his lips into an exaggerated kissing face, replete with the appropriate smacking sound. After each NP001 cycle, his speech also improved. He didn't always notice immediately, but friends and family would comment on how much easier he was to understand. And just like the first time, he could talk all day long without feeling fatigued. "Still sound like a drunk, but now I sound like a happy drunk," he told the forum.

One of the most dramatic effects Ben recorded while on NP001 was an increase in his hand strength. At the start of the trial, Ben's left hand tested in the 1st percentile. "That means 99% of forty-four year old males were stronger than me," he told the forum. For a former gymnast and rock climber, that was a bit of a punch to the gut. But after his third infusion, the strength in his left hand was average. "I can't stress enough just how monumental this is," he said.

He couldn't say for sure whether NP001 had improved his condition overall, but without a doubt it had stopped him from getting worse. "I was losing dexterity and strength in my left hand and left leg and, given another couple of months, my FRS score would have dropped 2–4 points. I have little doubt that NP001 prevented that." Instead, his FRS had held completely stable.

Rob enjoyed similar changes. In the middle of his second infusion cycle, he found that his swallowing was better and his tongue was stronger and had improved range of motion, allowing him to clear food from his cheeks. As with Ben, increased lip strength reduced Rob's drooling and restored his ability to pucker. In late June, he was even able to blow out his birthday candles, something he'd been unable to do the previous year. He also noticed increased range of motion in his right shoulder and neck, increased leg and arm strength, greater dexterity in his left hand, and improved leg coordination and balance. Among the side effects listed in his review of NP001 on PatientsLikeMe, he wrote: "Frequent smiling due to amazement over unanticipated improvement!"

Ben knew it was premature, but it certainly seemed like this drug had remarkable benefits—at least for some patients. People who had been suffering from ALS for many years and had been around the drug-development block a few times were cynical about Ben's enthusiasm. They had experienced the thrill of early-stage excitement many times before, and then the bitter aftertaste of a late-stage failure that always seemed to follow. But Ben was insistent. "There's more promise with this trial than there has been in the entire history of ALS," he told the *San Francisco Business Times* in September.[8] If broadcasting that information "comes at the risk of getting someone's hopes up," he added, "it is a risk worth taking."

"So, let me repeat," he concluded his forum post one morning. "NP001 stopped my ALS and it will probably stop yours."

Photos courtesy of the Harris family

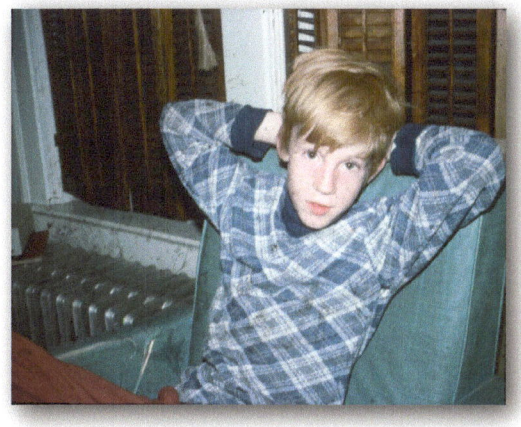

As a boy, in his home in Watertown, New York

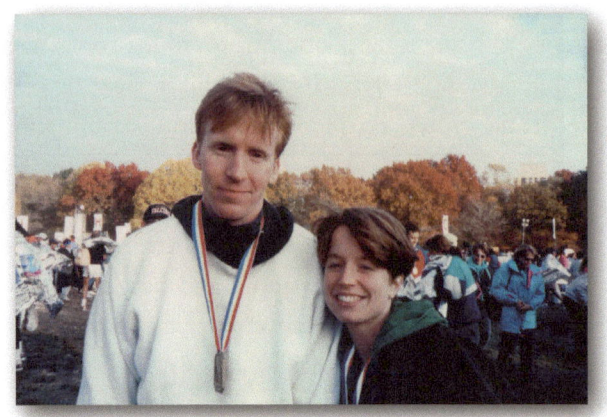

With wife Beccy, after completing the
NY Marathon in the early 1990s

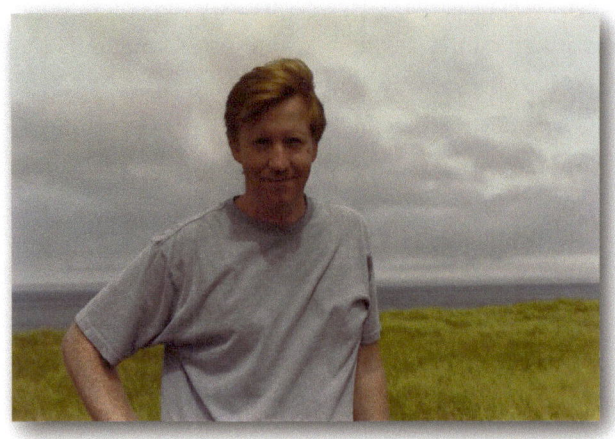

On vacation in Provincetown, Massachusetts, 1995

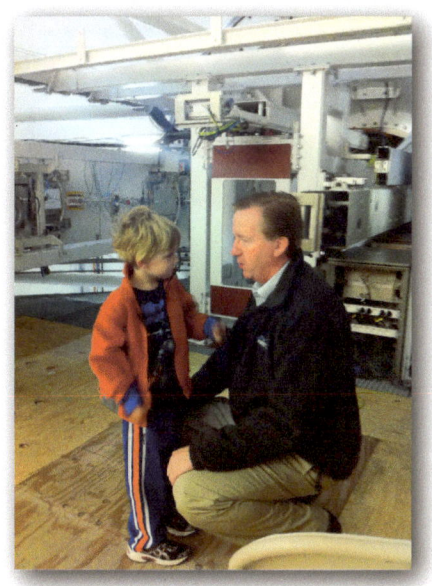

With son Rawden at a Proton Center
in Oklahoma City, 2009

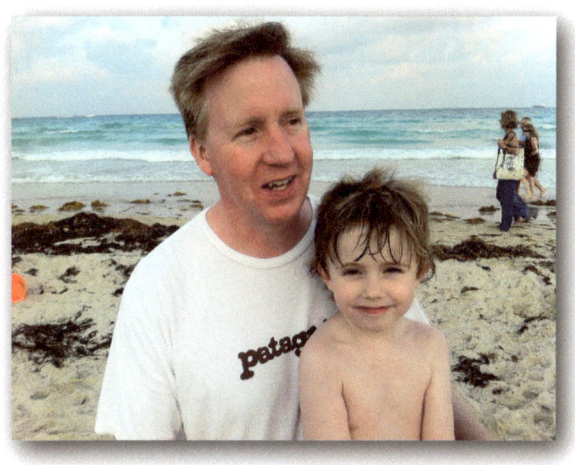

On vacation in Treasure Island, Florida, summer 2011

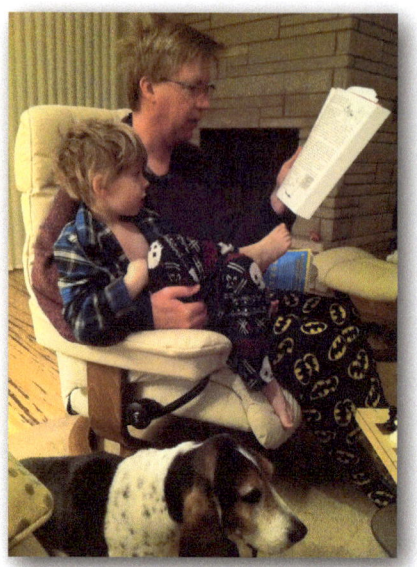

Reading with son Rawden and dog Otis, 2011

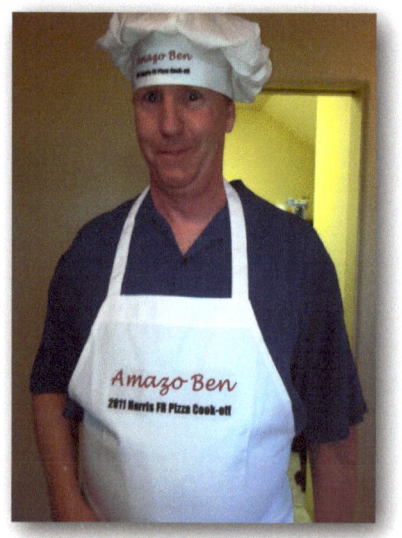

Participating in a pizza cook off at the Harris family reunion in Sedona, Arizona, 2011

Personal Trials

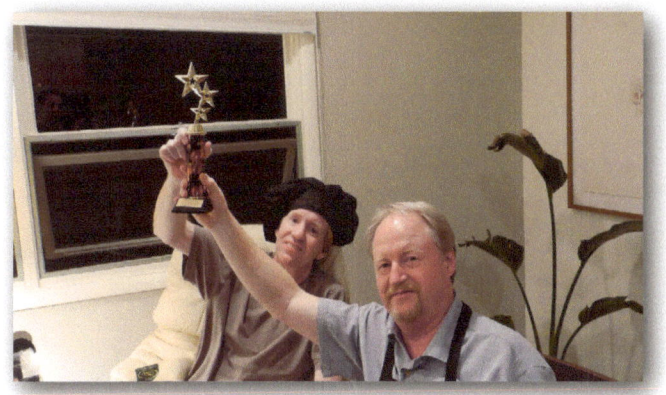

With brother Mike, holding up pizza cook off trophy
in Ben's home in Bloomington, Indiana, 2013

Five

DIY MEDICINE

The Phase 2 trial was double-blind, meaning that neither the patients nor their doctors were told which treatment group each participant had been assigned to. For good reason, participants hope to avoid the placebo group, but the FDA requires a placebo control to guard against the chance that participants' expectations of improvement will affect the results.

Despite the blinded nature of the study, both Rob and Ben believed they were on the drug as soon as they started to feel their bodies respond. They couldn't attribute the recovery of strength and motor control that they'd experienced to placebo effects; all they'd known since their diagnosis was decline. But Rob wanted to be sure. So he decided to swipe his IV bag from a trash bin at the Duke clinic and run a pH test on the residual solution inside. Rob was paired with two other ALS patients for his monthly infusions, a man about six years older than him and a woman who looked to be in her early sixties. The patients were escorted to a room with three cots, where they each received an IV drip—either a low or high dose of NP001, or saline.

Across the hall, their spouses chatted in a waiting area; the patients would join them after their infusions had finished while the medical staff continued to monitor them.

One afternoon, shortly after joining Kelly in the waiting room, Rob announced that he was feeling tired and headed back to his cot to rest. But he didn't lie down. Instead, he collected the used IV bags from the trash cans by each bed and tucked them in his iPad case, noting their order so he'd know which belonged to whom. Back at the hotel, he had Kelly cut the bags open and place a pH test strip inside each one. Within seconds, he knew who was getting which treatment. He was not surprised to learn that he was getting the high dose.

But Rob knew that didn't prove anything about the drug's effectiveness. His story was still just an anecdote. Only more data could reveal whether the drug was really working. He and Ben encouraged trial participants to record their progress on PatientsLikeMe; any and all data would be helpful, they said. Ben even suggested that patients get a hand dynamometer to test their grip—that's how he'd measured his dramatic increase in hand strength. If enough study participants tracked their data, Ben and Rob hoped to draw meaningful conclusions about how NP001 affected ALS.

The problem was, trial coordinators had only enrolled half the number of patients they needed to fill the study. "They hope to have full enrollment by September but at this rate this is optimistic," Ben told the others in mid-July. That was a serious concern. Taking extra time to fill the trial would delay the study's completion and the release of the results. This in turn would push back the possible launch of an expanded access program and additional clinical trials. "The longer it takes, the more people will die," Ben told the *San Francisco Business Times*.[9]

Rob emailed Neuraltus to have them update the list of participating medical centers on the study's clinicaltrials.gov page, while Ben worked on a way to get their story in the press. He wrote to Roger Ebert, who in March had given a TED Talk on what it means to lose one's voice.[9] Ben hoped that the movie critic might know someone who could help them raise awareness for the trial. Ben also queried the forum for anyone with contacts in the NFL who might draw a spotlight. A forum member who was friends with Montel Williams reached out to see what publicity the talk-show host could garner for the group. "The single most important task for us as a group is to fill this trial," Ben said.

It took a couple of months, but in the end their efforts paid off. In September, the company announced that it had filled the trial; Ben and Rob's advocacy had led to the enrollment of at least half a dozen patients. And in the end, more than thirty study participants—roughly one-third of all the patients involved in the NP001 trial—shared information about their disease on PatientsLikeMe.

To make sense of the data, Rob divided the patients into presumed treatment groups based on self-reported side effects, which included increased twitching, headaches, and fatigue. Rob knew it was an imperfect system for determining how much drug the patients had received, but those on the drug tended to experience worse side effects, and he figured it was as good a solution as any until patients were told which treatment group they'd been in. Then, using the FRS scores that patients had recorded on their PatientsLikeMe profiles, Rob compared the rate of disease progression between the two treatment groups and the placebo controls.

In his preliminary analysis, which Eric posted on his blog in January 2012, Rob found a statistically significant difference in the rate of disease progression between patients on the drug and those in the placebo group.[10] "This would be unprecedented for a Phase 2 ALS clinical trial," he wrote. The results of the Phase 2 trial of dexpramipexole had been announced just a couple months earlier, and they were not even close to statistical significance, Rob noted; more like statistically *suggestive*. The main part of the study, which compared ALS progression over twelve weeks in patients taking one of three doses of dex with those taking a placebo, yielded a statistical p-value of 0.11, meaning there was a greater than 10% likelihood the results were due to chance. Scientific standard typically demands a p-value of less than 0.05 for the coveted claim of statistical significance. Nevertheless, the study was considered a success, and the drug's developers were already enrolling patients in a large Phase 3 trial (the study Ben had nearly chosen to join instead of NP001). Rob hoped that the statistically significant result yielded by his analysis of the PatientsLikeMe data would also be reflected in Neuraltus's analysis of the real trial data, prompting the FDA to consider accelerated approval for NP001.

While the drug's continued progress from bench to bedside would be good news for all ALS patients, Rob's analysis also fueled the forum's quest for an alternative option for those unable to participate in the trial. WF10 still seemed like a promising lead, and was readily available from Thailand, but the circumstances were dubious at best, and the cost was prohibitive for most, including Eric. Some forum members learned of a special access program in Canada that could supply WF10, but it required a prescription from a Canadian physician, something that no one could seem to get. It wasn't long before some patients began to consider a third, more radical, possibility: plain sodium chlorite, the chemical the patients now knew to be the active ingredient of both NP001 and WF10. It was commonly used in low concentrations for water purification, and it could be purchased from online suppliers for just $50 a quart.

"Chlorite is chlorite," said Ben. "If the chlorite ion is doing the work of NP001, it doesn't really matter how it gets into the blood."

Of course, most patients did not have the proper equipment or training to set up an intravenous infusion to deliver the chemical as NP001 or WF10 was given—nor were they comfortable injecting themselves with a store-bought chemical of unknown purity. But many seemed open to ingesting it. After all, various forms of chlorite had been marketed as dietary supplements, and the chemical was used in food processing, in addition to both commercial and personal water treatment.

The big question was whether sodium chlorite that was ingested would make it to the blood, where it could flip the switch to make macrophages stop promoting inflammation—and thus killing neurons—and start cleaning up the mess. The first stop in the gastrointestinal tract, the stomach, contains acids that aid digestion, and acids trigger a reaction that converts sodium chlorite to another chemical called chlorine dioxide, a powerful bleaching agent at high concentrations. The forum members turned to the literature on water purification to learn what they could about this process, but whether the stomach acid would prevent sodium chlorite from reaching the blood remained unclear.

Then, Eric got an email from a chemist named Tom Poast. *There are ways to safely ingest sodium chlorite,* Tom told him. *Oral consumption can get chlorite into your system.*

In 2007, a few years before Neuraltus launched its Phase 1 trial for NP001, Tom Poast's wife had handed him a book by a man named Jim Humble on something called Miracle Mineral Supplement (MMS), a solution Humble marketed as 28% sodium chlorite. Humble claimed that the product had successfully treated all sorts of ailments, from AIDS to cancer, and that it had cured more than seventy-five thousand cases of malaria. The 28% chlorite solution was

Personal Trials

intended to be diluted and mixed with an "activator," some kind of acid that would convert the sodium chlorite into chlorine dioxide. In addition to serving as the key player in water purification, chlorine dioxide had been rumored to fight disease by increasing oxygen delivery to the cells of the body.

Tom, who worked as a test engineer for Structural Diagnostic Testing Services in Bellingham, Washington, had been exposed to similar supplements before. He'd grown up watching his parents take products marketed as "stabilized oxygen" to treat various aches and pains. His dad would take the little brown bottle out of the cupboard and use an eyedropper to deliver a few drops into a small glass of water, then guzzle the drink. So when Tom's wife gave him Jim Humble's book on MMS, he read it with an open mind. But the more he learned, the more skeptical he became. The advertised concentration of 28% seemed dangerous—most stabilized oxygen products had just a 2–5% concentration of chlorite—and something wasn't right with Humble's calculations for how to dilute and activate the mixture prior to ingestion. Humble claimed that his MMS preparation would create a solution that contained less than 1 milligram of chlorine dioxide per liter; Tom calculated a much different number: around 300 milligrams per liter, or three hundred times the Environmental Protection Agency-recommended levels. *This is the craziest thing I've ever heard of,* Tom recalled thinking after he finished reading the book. "Jim is a great storyteller, but he doesn't have a clue when it comes to chemistry," he said later.*

Tom would know. For more than thirty years he'd run nondestructive experiments on building products like piping and storage tanks. He'd tested how various chemicals, including sodium chlorite,

---

* In 2010, the FDA warned consumers against ingesting MMS. "The product, when used as directed, produces an industrial bleach that can cause serious harm to health," the agency wrote.

affected the integrity of the vessels used to store and transport them, making sure they didn't cause any corrosion. Sodium chlorite was also a tool Tom often pulled from his trusty chemistry set at home. After a big meal of freshly caught Dungeness crab—a luxury of living near the coast in Washington State—the shells in the trash would soon begin to waft an overwhelming stench. "You can smell the garbage can from a block away," Tom said. So he mixed up a little sodium chlorite and hydrochloric acid, and voilà: the odor would vanish. "With the right chemical treatment, you can remove the cause and not just cover it up." Tom had also mixed sodium chlorite and citric acid powders to zap the musty stench from old cars, and stubborn pet odors that had permeated the seats of an old van. Tom even had experience using sodium chlorite as a disinfectant, and often included it in a Boy Scouts course he taught on water purification.

And so, despite the flaws he had identified in Humble's approach, Tom didn't totally discount the possibility that a chlorite solution could be beneficial to health. He decided to order some MMS to do a little testing of his own. He experimented with diluting the sodium chlorite in some of the drinking buckets his friends put out for their animals. Tom would calculate a low concentration that he thought could help prevent the formation of slime around the edges of the water bowl. Then, unexpectedly, Tom began to notice the animals perking up. They had more energy and appeared less stiff. He recalled one time when he and his friend miscalculated the volume of the drinking bucket and accidentally dosed a group of dogs with a higher concentration than intended. The result was shocking. An old dog named Max, who rarely got up except to eat and use the bathroom, was suddenly running around the yard with the younger dogs and leaping unassisted into the van for road trips. "That made me focus," Tom said.

He posted updates about his experiments on the online message board CureZone, and soon people were contacting him about how to use sodium chlorite to treat their cows, horses, chickens, and llamas. Some even expressed interest in taking it for their own maladies, and they would come to Tom for advice. He'd emphasize that this was an unproven treatment, and that caution was vital when dealing with these chemicals, but he couldn't turn away from the patients' desperate calls for help. "Without going into details, we have seen wonderful improvements with many diseases," Tom said, including various infections, malaria, and some cancers. Tom even guided people who'd had success in treating their multiple sclerosis, a neurodegenerative disease of the central nervous system, like ALS. "There was a group of fifteen or twenty people trying it for various things," Tom recalled. "My job, if you will, was to try and make scientific sense of it."

The home remedies didn't work for everyone, Tom said, but many used sodium chlorite regularly, and it appeared to cause no serious harm. Tom couldn't explain the biology supporting its effects, but the evidence was hard to ignore. "It was enough that when this ALS thing came up I thought, well, we've got a reasonable chance."

Tom came across the ALS forum in early summer 2011 while searching the web for new data on sodium chlorite that might inform his Boy Scouts water purification course. At first, Tom hesitated to get involved, wary of leading desperate patients down a rabbit hole. He had no clinical proof that chlorite would help, and there were no studies to rule out long-term side effects. "I'm not a medical professional, so who the hell am I to say, 'Drink this bleach chemical'?" he said.

But he had lost a friend to ALS just a few months earlier, and he regretted not having introduced him to sodium chlorite before it was too late. And the patients on the forums were clearly informed and competent. He decided to share what he knew about the chemical, and let the patients make their own decisions about how to use the information. "I thought, I have a little bit of knowledge here, and I'm not afraid to throw my hat in the ring," Tom said. He reached out to Eric, who connected him with Ben and Rob. With their encouragement, Tom began posting on the forum.

He emphasized caution. In contrast to both WF10 and NP001, there were no human trials on sodium chlorite. "Anecdotally, a lot of people have ingested chlorite solutions and they aren't dead, but that doesn't mean that it is safe," he said. And he couldn't answer the group's question about ingested chlorite making it to where it might stave off further neurodegeneration—he was a chemist, not a biologist—but it seemed possible to him. "A solution taken orally doesn't have to deal with the blood chemistry, and chlorite ends up in all the organs of the body, including the brain," he wrote to the forum in mid-July. "At least this is the case with animals, but there is no indication that it works any differently in humans." There was reason for hope, and for some unable to try WF10 or NP001, the potential could outweigh the risk.

Eric concluded that it did. After reading all the safety studies on sodium chlorite that he could find, Eric reasoned that ingesting a chlorite solution was unlikely to do serious harm. And it was cheap, so there was no financial risk. On August 10, 2011, Eric had his mom administer his first dose into his feeding tube—1 liter of sodium chlorite–spiked water mainlined to his stomach.

After five days of this, Eric recorded his first positive effect in his openly shared patient log: "Seemingly clearer speech." Similar to Ben's and Rob's experiences on NP001, Eric noticed some mild fatigue following the treatment. He also experienced some loose stool, which he had known was a possible side effect. But he did seem to feel a little better. "I haven't jumped out of bed, but I have felt more robust," Eric said after his second treatment cycle. After another few cycles, he uploaded a video showing his improved limb strength. While seated, he was able to rock his knee, which was extremely slender from lack of musculature, from left to right by several inches, and he could stop or start his leg at any point. His mom couldn't stop repeating "wow" as she held the camera.

In addition to logging his progress, Eric set to work building a website to host information and results relating to sodium chlorite. In September he shared the site with the group and invited others who chose to take sodium chlorite to track their outcomes. The site also offered background information on sodium chlorite and detailed instructions to help interested patients follow the protocol. Eric even embedded a dosage calculator to determine specific preparations based on body weight. The effort was researched, organized, and structured. If sodium chlorite worked, the group wanted to demonstrate that with data—apples-to-apples data—and not just their individual success stories.

It wasn't the first time the ALS community had initiated a do-it-yourself (DIY) clinical trial to test an unproven treatment on themselves. In November 2007, researchers in Italy reported the results of a small trial in which sixteen ALS patients took doses of lithium carbonate, an approved drug for bipolar disorder.[11] Twenty-eight additional patients served as placebo controls. According to the scientists, the treatment significantly slowed disease progression, and none of the patients taking lithium died during the fifteen-month trial.

Unfortunately, no one seemed to be planning a follow-up study. Lithium is a natural compound and not itself patentable, so perhaps there wasn't money in such a venture. Whatever the reason, ALS patients chatting online began to discuss the possibility of trying lithium outside the context of an FDA-sanctioned clinical trial. It was already on the market for bipolar disorder, so all they needed was a doctor who was willing to write them a prescription for its off-label use.

Several people contacted the Italian group to get the dose, while others dug up what they could on lithium's safety. Humberto Macedo, an ALS patient in Brazil, started a Google Docs spreadsheet for recording data, and Karen Felzer, a geophysicist whose father had ALS, built a website to host the results and share information about the treatment. By May 2008, nearly two hundred ALS patients had signed up for the experiment, including Eric.

Unfortunately, lithium ultimately proved unsuccessful in curtailing ALS progression. After about four months, Eric and most of the others saw no effects; some patients even reported that their decline had quickened. Karen used her background in statistics—normally devoted to analyzing earthquake aftershocks—to evaluate the data and confirmed the disappointment: there was no evidence that lithium slowed FRS decline. An analysis by researchers at PatientsLikeMe of the data reported on their site[12] and more than one official clinical trial[13] eventually came to the same conclusion: lithium does not help ALS patients, and may even accelerate the disease.

"The lithium project was the first example showing that people around the world could organize, accept a protocol, stick to it, and reliably report results," Eric said. Even though the treatment itself wasn't successful, the DIY trial was, he said. And, importantly, they'd made their efforts public. Countless clinical trials that yield such negative findings are never even published, meaning that the biomedical research community could waste time and resources—and, potentially, patients' lives—repeating past mistakes.

Personal Trials

Obviously, the ALS patients taking sodium chlorite were hoping for a different outcome than the lithium experiment, but regardless of their personal gain, most felt strongly about sharing data on their progress so that, whatever happened, the effort would not go to waste. Two months after Eric launched the chlorite project website, more than a dozen other ALS patients had started logging their progress as they dosed themselves with the homemade remedy. And the first reports sounded generally promising.

A fellow member of Ben's ALS support group in Bloomington posted that he was feeling "definite improvements with both leg strength and arm/hand strength." Several patients also reported improvements to their voice, changes that were noticed by their friends and family. Others said that swallowing fluids was suddenly easier, and caused less choking and coughing. A woman in the UK had improved leg strength and slightly restored mobility in her right hand after taking sodium chlorite; another patient's right foot and toes were flexing more easily.

Ben couldn't contain himself. "I'm getting goosebumps," he said. "This stuff might really work!!"

Six

On their own

As Ben's and Rob's NP001 treatments went on, a pattern became clear: they would feel a little better for a couple of weeks, then slowly regress until they got their next round of the drug. They knew that if they didn't get extra infusions after the trial, the decline they experienced in between treatments would continue indefinitely, as it had before the study had begun.

Even if the company did offer an expanded access program after the Phase 2 trial was complete, that wouldn't start for at least a few months after their last infusions. Part of the trial protocol included a three-month observation period, which the patients suspected was to record the resumption of disease progression, as well as any change in the biomarkers the researchers were tracking. Each month, as they traveled to their trial sites, Rob and Ben were confronted with the reality that their treatments would soon be finished, at least for a few months and possibly forever. To not be able to continue was "cruel," Ben wrote to the forum in September. "After six infusion cycles we will die."

Both men continued to religiously record their progress on PatientsLikeMe. They were hopeful that researchers at Neuraltus would see how much they were improving on the drug and allow them to continue NP001 infusions without interruption. Rob noted that the dexpramipexole trial had offered open-label extension for those in the trial. "This is a win-win situation when the drug is deemed safe and shows some benefit," Rob told the group. "It provides further, longer term safety data and efficacy data as well. I really hope Neuraltus Pharmaceuticals will reconsider this."

In late 2011, an ALS patient advocacy group known as ALS Treat Us Now launched a petition calling for any ALS drug that has shown safety and efficacy in a Phase 2 trial to be made available, specifically naming NP001 and dex. The petition eventually amassed more than eighteen thousand supporters, but, as Neuraltus sought funding for a Phase 3 trial, the company did not offer an expanded access program.

In desperation, Rob began to make his personal case for continued treatment. If he could demonstrate his exceptional response to the drug, there was no way the company could deny him access. The drug was stopping his disease, and without it, he would die. He compiled charts of his progress, illustrating how his rapid decline had not only ceased but actually reversed during his time on NP001. Over the past few months, his FRS score had gone from 35 to 38; if he had continued to progress at the same rate he had prior to the trial, his score would have dropped to 29.

Rob shared the information with Dr. Bedlack, who agreed that he had a strong case. Of all the NP001 trial participants that Dr. Bedlack had observed, Rob had benefited as much as anyone. "His speech became a lot more clear; the movement in his limbs became more useful," Dr. Bedlack said later. "Up until that point, that was probably one of the first patients I ever saw dramatically improve, either spontaneously or in the course of a clinical trial."

Dr. Bedlack appealed to Neuraltus on Rob's behalf, but he knew the company was unlikely to grant any patient continued NP001 treatments. At a meeting before the trial had even begun, Neuraltus executives had explained to Dr. Bedlack and other study investigators that infusions would not be available following the trial. Later on, as requests for continued access started to roll in, the execs sent around talking points that offered guidance to the researchers on how to discuss this very issue with patients who asked. The company simply couldn't afford it. The actual cost to produce the drug for an expanded access program was prohibitive for the small firm, and allowing continued treatments on an individual basis was risky. Neuraltus had to focus on getting the drug to market, where it could benefit a far greater number of patients.

Sure enough, Neuraltus declined Dr. Bedlack's request. Dr. Bedlack called to share the bad news, but Rob had known it was coming. And he was already plotting his alternative chlorite treatment.

Before his last infusion cycle late that fall, Ben ordered a small supply of WF10—fifty vials, or enough for five rounds of infusions. He paid $14,000, including shipping from Thailand. But knowing his family wouldn't be able to afford it for very long—a year's supply would top $60,000—he also ordered a quart of sodium chlorite from an online site called Keavy's Corner for just $50. It would last him fifteen years at the dosage outlined in the patients' protocol.

Ben decided that he would wait as long as possible before trying one of the two alternative forms of chlorite. He was still serving as a data point for the trial and he didn't want to compromise the results. If he started taking an alternative form of chlorite, and it worked, it could misleadingly suggest to trial investigators that NP001 had an enduring effect—when he and Rob knew all too well that the drug's benefit was only temporary.

Ben got his last infusions of NP001 the second week of November. By that time, he was easily fatigued, but he felt in better shape than he had before he started the trial. He was still mobile, could drive himself around, and even worked full time. But by mid-December, Ben's body was fielding new assaults. "Salivation is at this point worse than it was pre-NP001. I have to work hard not to drool while I eat," he wrote in a review of NP001 on his PatientsLikeMe profile.

After all the progress he'd made during the trial, to regress was heartrending. Over the next few weeks, his left leg weakened and threw his gait off balance. His speech and swallowing also declined considerably. "I now have to drink water in very small sips to prevent myself from choking and I find that I am having difficulty swallowing food, even choking on occasion. It feels to me that my progression has now picked up where it left off just before I started the NP001 infusions."

He decided to put off trying an alternative form of chlorite until the new year. This could very well be the last Christmas he'd spend with Beccy and their son; for now, he just wanted to enjoy his family. He and Rawden constructed a 3-D printer from a kit, finishing just a few days before Santa Claus arrived. It was a nice, quiet holiday.

But by early January, he couldn't wait any longer. He mixed up the oral dose of sodium chlorite as described on the website Eric had built, and sipped down two rounds. He waited anxiously for the rejuvenation he'd enjoyed after each round of NP001, but none came. Guessing it was because ingesting the chlorite solution wasn't delivering enough of the chemical to his bloodstream, where it could work its magic, he wasted no time in moving to WF10 infusions. As a physician's assistant, Beccy had experience with inserting a peripheral line.

On January 19, she set Ben up in the living room, in his favorite recliner on the far side of the couch with a good view of the TV, the kitchen, and the front door. He settled in and watched the solution drip into his blood, just like the NP001 had, and once again waited for his limbs to strengthen and his speech and swallowing to improve.

But once again, he was disappointed. "After two days of WF10 I don't feel any better than after two days of oral sodium chlorite," he posted on the forum. Over the next few days, he noticed slight improvements, but nothing happened that might justify the massive price tag. "I was surprised; I thought there would be a big difference between WF10 and oral sodium chlorite, but there really wasn't."

Since he'd bought the stuff, Ben decided to stick with WF10 for a while, completing three five-day courses. But save a few minor improvements, the treatment did not deliver the effects that he'd enjoyed during the NP001 trial. But before he gave up on sodium chlorite entirely, Ben decided to try one last option—an injection of a pure sodium chlorite solution. WF10 was only part chlorite; it also contained a compound called sodium chlor*ate*. NP001, by contrast, was all chlorite. Ingesting chlorite hadn't been effective, but if he could prep the sodium chlorite he'd bought online to safely inject into his vein, perhaps that would come the closest to mimicking the NP001 infusions. He believed the 5% sodium chlorite he'd bought from Keavy's Corner was sterile; he just needed to figure out the proper dilution to create a dose that would be equivalent to his NP001 treatments. "I am still convinced we can do this," he told the group. "Of course you have to be absolutely insane to try this. Which I am."

Others voiced concerns about the safety of the approach, including Tom, who recalled offering "every caution I could without standing right in his way." But as Ben's body continued to fail him, he decided it was worth a shot. On March 14, he set up his infusion. He'd recently had a port installed to easily tap into his bloodstream, so he didn't need Beccy's help this time. He hooked up the sodium chlorite solution himself and waited as it dripped into his body.

At first, he didn't notice any effect. Perhaps chlorite—in any form—was only a short-term fix. Even NP001 had seemed less and less effective over the course of the trial. But after his second round of sodium chlorite infusions, he got a pleasant surprise: he was once again able to drink water—without effort and without choking.

Ben was watching Rawden on the rope swing in their backyard when, without thinking about it, he grabbed his glass of seltzer and took a sip. After a few minutes, he realized that the bubbly beverage had gone flat. Yet he was having no trouble drinking it. It had been more than a month since he'd been able to drink uncarbonated water; he found it much harder to swallow than seltzer or milk. But that day, watching his son swing, the flat seltzer went down without a hitch. "The difference is small but unquestionably real," he wrote in his review of sodium chlorite on PatientsLikeMe. "This is very encouraging and tells me that chlorite is still having some effect."

Unfortunately, with the exception of one more slight reprieve of symptoms that summer when he could hold his head above water during a swimming class, the effects continued to wane. By the time the Harris family met in Sedona for their next reunion, Ben relied heavily on a cane. He was unable to hike to the top of Cathedral Rock; he could barely make it down to the nearby creek.

Seven

Learning to die

Rob was wary of the sodium chlorite route. But he was interested in trying WF10 and Ben agreed to share his supply. In February 2012, Rob headed down to Florida to stay with his parents while his cousin, a nurse, helped him set up the infusions. Immediately, Rob noticed some minor changes, similar to the benefits he gained from his NP001 treatments. His speech and swallowing improved, and his hands uncurled, becoming more flexible and dexterous. His balance, speed, and ability to lift his feet also got noticeably better, and he was able to walk without his cane for the first time in months.

But the improvements were short-lived, and in the end they were not as significant as they had been on NP001. Besides, there was no way Rob could afford to get a steady supply of WF10. His family had already sacrificed enough for this damned disease, having lost the mountain house that he and Kelly had helped build. He wasn't about to embark on a misguided attempt to save his own life only to leave them with nothing. He'd finish up the WF10 Ben had sent, but until

Neuraltus reconsidered an expanded access program, that would be the end of his chlorite treatments.

When he returned home three weeks later, his disease came roaring back, just as Ben had experienced. At the time of his WF10 infusions in February, Rob recorded an FRS score of 30 on PatientsLikeMe. His little icon had a green torso, yellow head and legs, and orange arms and hands. By June, all but his torso was orange, and Rob's FRS had dropped to 19—a score lower than many patients have when they die. Rob rarely left his electric wheelchair, often choosing to sleep in it because of how much he hated the complete immobility he felt when transferred to the bed.

His declining ability to communicate compounded the loss of his independence. One time he was so frustrated that he got out his iPad to show Kelly a diagram of the human jaw, to explain how she was missing some of his teeth when she brushed them. Rob was humiliated that he'd become such a strain on the family, and he withdrew. Leaving the house had become too much of a hassle anyway, so he simply stopped going to Sydne's gymnastics meets and to Tyler's soccer games. Kelly was forced to take on a full-time job to pay the bills, and when she wasn't at work or shuttling the kids around, she was feeding Rob or cleaning up after him. Kelly was exhausted. Rob was angry. The routine tasks of everyday life took up all their time, and there simply wasn't any left over to just curl up and love each other.

But in the ALS community, Rob wasn't the useless cripple he sometimes believed himself to be at home; he was a hero. He devoted nearly all his time to researching the disease, discussing possible mechanisms and treatments with other patients on the forums, and participating in other ALS-related projects. He worked with researchers at the Centers for Disease Control and Prevention to help establish the National ALS Registry and served as a clinical research ambassador for the Northeast ALS Consortium, helping to educate ALS patients about clinical trials and to drive enrollment. In May, he was presented with the Rasmussen

Advocate of the Year Award "for his persistent efforts to encourage others living with ALS like him to follow his lead by embracing advocacy and public policy as a means to find a treatment and cure."

At the end of August, Tyler had a soccer tournament down in South Carolina. Kelly and Rob's twin sister Cassie, who was in town from Michigan, were thrilled when Rob said he wanted to go. They loaded up the van and hit the road for the three-hour drive. The ride was hard on Rob, though; he found it hard to get comfortable. And his one outlet for exercising his own free will—his wheelchair—was locked in place in the center of the van. On his iPad, he typed a message to Cassie, saying that he was too hot; she turned the air conditioning up. Then Rob said he was cold, so she turned it back down. A few minutes later, Rob asked Cassie to turn the music down—it was too loud. Cassie obliged. But as the complaints kept coming, she couldn't suppress her annoyance. *Will you stop?!* she snapped.

With tempers wearing thin, Rob didn't feel like gathering with the players and their parents for take-out from Carrabba's Italian Grill after the first round of games on Saturday. He sent Kelly and Tyler off to the party, while Cassie stayed with him back at the hotel. He was visibly upset. It wasn't his fault his body was failing him; why wasn't his family more understanding? Everything had just become too hard. *I don't want to live like this anymore*, he told his sister.

"We take for granted that, the radio's too loud, you turn it down; you can't hear it, you turn it up; you're too hot, you adjust," Cassie said later. "He couldn't do anything, so he's at our mercy." The car ride had made it all too clear to Rob, who had been an athlete and avid outdoorsman, just how limited his life had become. Cassie wasn't ready to lose her brother just yet, and she told him as much. But Rob had made up his mind, and Cassie knew she had to respect his choice. She told him that she and her husband would look into planning a trip to Switzerland, where patients could get help ending their own lives.

Personal Trials

The next morning, the family dropped Tyler with his team before taking Rob for some breakfast. He wanted MacDonald's pancakes. There was a Burger King near the soccer fields, but that wouldn't do, he said—it had to be MacDonald's. "I think we drove 20 miles to find those pancakes," said Cassie. She again felt annoyed that Rob, who couldn't even feed himself, was being so damn particular about something as meaningless as where they went for breakfast. But she knew how much food had come to matter to him; with only so many meals left, they had better be whatever he was craving. When they finally found a Mickey D's, Rob told Cassie to get him two orders of hotcakes. Kelly cut them up and fed them to him until he'd had his fill. That was the last meal he ever ate.

Rob knew the Switzerland trip was a pipe dream; the logistics would be a nightmare, never mind the cost. And he didn't want to wait. He had decided that he would stop eating. Back at home on Monday morning, Rob had Cassie call the florist. If he was going to die in the very near future, he had a few things he needed to get in order. Kelly's birthday was the following week, and he wanted her to have a dozen red roses. And Tyler was about to turn sixteen—he would need a candy bouquet. And of course sweet Sydne, who the following March would be turning thirteen, a teenager! He had Cassie order her a dozen roses as well. Finally, he tacked on an order for his and Kelly's next anniversary; it would be eighteen years. "Rob just thought of it all," Cassie said. She, Rob, and the woman at the flower shop sobbed as Cassie placed the orders.

On Tuesday, Rob went to Sydne's gymnastics class. On Thursday night, it was Tyler's soccer game. He knew it would be the last time he ever saw his kids run. That weekend, hospice came to the house, and the waiting began. When Kelly's flowers arrived on her birthday the following Wednesday, Rob was still conscious to see her receive them. Later that night, he slipped into a coma and slept for two days straight. On Friday, he woke up briefly to find himself surrounded by family. He looked at the nine people around him and labored a "Hi" to each. Then he slipped back into unconsciousness, this time forever.

On the night of Sunday, September 9, 2012, Kelly and Cassie lay in bed next to Rob, who was in his wheelchair. Kelly had dozed off, but Cassie was still awake, listening for Rob's next breath. Then, a little after 4 a.m., she didn't hear it. She woke up Kelly, then her parents. Rob was gone.

"He would never say, 'I died of ALS,' " Cassie said. "He lived with ALS until he couldn't live anymore."

The ALS community mourned Rob's passing. Eric was hit especially hard. "Fuck fuck fuckity fucking fuck-all fuck fuck!" was the best way he could describe his reaction. Having dealt with ALS for nearly a decade, Eric had seen a lot of good people die. And while he understood there were limits to what some would do to survive, he remained hopeful that a successful treatment—maybe even NP001—was around the corner. "I honestly feel that the miracle is imminent," he said at the time. If only Rob had accepted a feeding tube and ventilator, he might have lived long enough for that to happen.

Ben, too, was gutted by Rob's death, but he saw a similar future for himself. He had decided from the beginning that the day he was unable to get to the kitchen to make himself a meal would be the day he stopped eating altogether. That day came in early August 2013, just under a year after Rob died.

After sodium chlorite failed to deliver improvements, Ben had tried numerous other experimental therapies. His PatientsLikeMe profile lists more than fifty interventions, including an experimental stem cell procedure in Alabama that seemed to briefly improve his muscle function. He also took a combination of three peptides that he ordered directly from a manufacturer after determining their structure from the scientific literature. But nothing made a significant difference in his decline, and in the end, everything just became too difficult. "takes me 5 minutes to ge tone sock on and I have to rest for 5 minutes after that," he struggled to type. "I don't sleep very well, wake up every half hour, legs usually in pain. I can't turn myself over very well, it feels like being burring alive. can't lie on back, I start choking on saliva, and when I lay on side my shoulder has no mucles and the bones grind against each other. it torture during the day andtorture all night. lung capacity is at 50%, i get out of breath whenever I move any part of my body."

Add to all his personal pain and suffering the hardship he was putting his family through, and Ben knew it was time to let go. He wanted Rawden to have a normal childhood, even if it had to be without a father, and he wanted Beccy to be able to move on with her own life, and not spend all her energy and love on him. The family planned one last reunion, this time in Ben's home in Bloomington. In March, big brother Mike sent out an email to everyone letting them know that by June it might be too late. Over the next couple of months, everyone made the trip.

On August 5, 2013, Ben stopped eating and drinking. He felt his body weaken immediately. The following day, he wrote a goodbye letter to his friends on the forum, expressing his gratitude for all the discussions and DIY experiments that had helped occupy his mind for the past two years. In the end, although his disease had progressed as predicted from the outset, he still considered his self-experimentation successful. He'd detailed everything so that present and future ALS patients could learn from his experiences.

"I can die knowing that I contributed to finding a treatment," he wrote on the forum. And then he repeated his mantra, which had defined the work of Eric, Rob, himself, and the rest of the group: "This above all else is the most important thing: *If it is done in secret, it is done in vain.*"

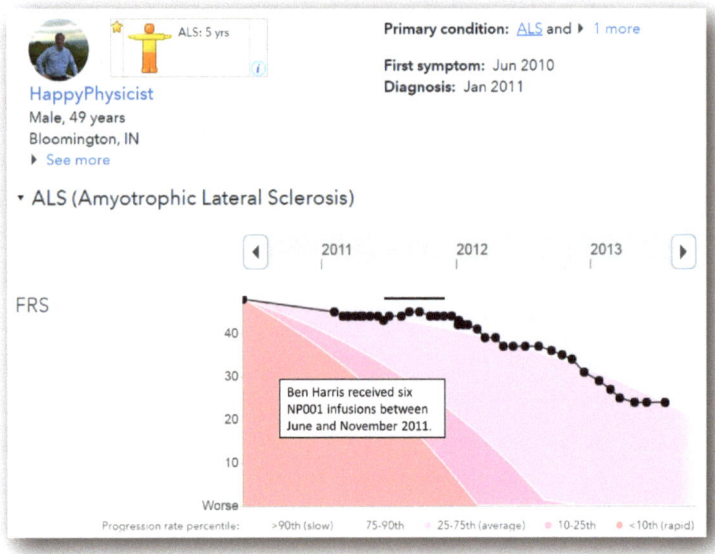

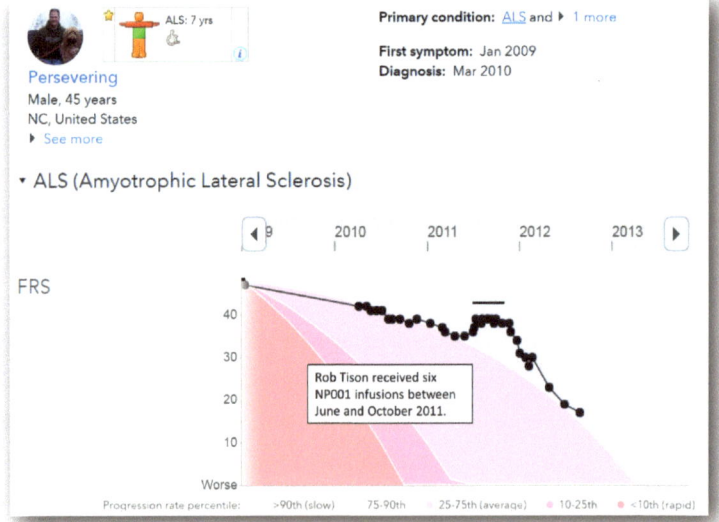

Both Ben Harris (HappyPhysicist) and Rob Tison (Persevering) made their PatientsLikeMe profiles public. You can explore their diseases and attempted treatments, and read their own notes about their experiments and their bodies' declines, at www.patientslikeme.com, where ALS patients continue to input new data every day.

Epilogue

Capitalizing on DIY medicine

> *Once upon a time we had a very paternalistic system, where patients would come, and they would have a set of symptoms, and doctors would ask all the questions and give all the answers. And in the past decade things have really shifted almost to the other side, where a lot of medicine is autonomous now. You see these DIY programs where patients are deciding, after doing an Internet search, that this is what they want to do; they go get the medicine, they take it, and they log their own output measures.*
>
> –Richard Bedlack, director of the
> Duke University ALS Clinic

April 24, 2012. Jamie Heywood stared at his computer screen, his focus trained on a graph depicting the progress of fourteen ALS patients who'd been ingesting sodium chlorite and reporting their progress on PatientsLikeMe. It was an ethical dilemma that Jamie hadn't foreseen when he'd started the creative and successful social media platform nearly eight years earlier. The patients taking the homemade remedy were, on average, declining at a slightly slower rate than a set of control patients that Jamie and his analysts had culled from the PatientsLikeMe database. But with so few patients and so much variation in their disease progression, Jamie couldn't say with confidence whether sodium chlorite was stalling ALS.

He was conflicted. Should he share the analysis with PatientsLikeMe members, some of whom were still ingesting doses of sodium chlorite? They were the ones who made it possible, after all, and ALS patients didn't have time to wait for research to deliver a more definitive answer. But he was confronted with the dangerous prospect that someone could misunderstand or misrepresent the results.

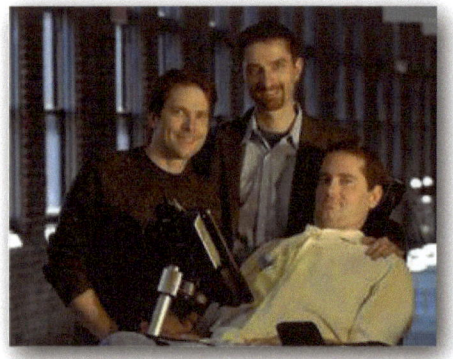

Jamie (left), Ben (middle), and Stephen Heywood, May 2006
PHOTO BY RICHARD HOWARD

"I'm looking at fourteen patients and an effect that's a third the size of an error bar, so I know there's not a dramatic difference. But you could remake this graph, and people would believe the data in a very different way," he tells me over the phone. "And so the scientific methodology is morally unacceptable from a human rights standpoint, and the release of the data as it stands might produce harm because it will be misinterpreted."

In addition to the moral responsibility, whether to share the data was a personal decision for Jamie. In the late 1990s, his younger brother Stephen, who was just twenty-nine, was diagnosed with ALS,

Personal Trials

and Jamie had spent the better part of his professional life working to discover a cure.

Late one evening in December 1998, Jamie was in his office at the Neurosciences Institute in La Jolla, California, when he received a call from Stephen. He'd recently accepted a position as the director of technology development at the persuasion of Nobel laureate Gerald Edelman, a neuroscience pioneer seeking to understand the human brain. Jamie wasn't a neuroscientist; he wasn't even a biologist. He was an MIT-trained engineer. But when Edelman invited Jamie to help him "commercialize the biological basis of consciousness," the opportunity was too sexy to turn down, Jamie recalls.

He'd been with the institute for less than a year when his brother called to tell him he had ALS. Jamie put in his notice the next morning, preparing to move back to the East Coast to be with his family. But Jamie didn't leave right away. He recognized the potential advantage of his newfound position in the neuroscience community, and so he stayed for two months under the tutelage of his scientific colleagues, including the Nobel laureate himself. Jamie learned everything he could about genetics, neurons, neurodegeneration, and ALS. Then, in February, he and his wife packed up their lives in Southern California and drove the three thousand miles to Boston, where Jamie and Stephen would start a nonprofit biotech company to expedite the search for a cure. Somewhere in the middle of Oklahoma, in a moving truck that couldn't top fifty-five miles per hour, Jamie drafted a letter that defined his vision for the company, called the ALS Therapy Development Foundation (later, the ALS Therapy Development

Institute, or ALS TDI). "My brain switched," he said. "It went out of learn mode into execution mode."

One treatment that Jamie ushered through preclinical research was a stem cell transplant that Stephen, along with two other patients, eventually received. "It was literally less than two years to go from the initial concept discussion through the validation experiments, rodent toxicology and safety, primate toxicology and safety, and then ultimately into my brother and other patients," Jamie said. Unfortunately, with only three anecdotes and no control, it was unclear whether the treatment had helped at all. It didn't seem to, and Jamie ultimately shuttered that line of inquiry, but he sometimes wondered if he'd made the right decision. The researchers needed a way to better assess these kinds of individual trials. Although they don't conform to traditional clinical research standards, with enough of them, surely it would be better than nothing.

In addition to evaluating the sanctioned experimental treatment of individual patients, Jamie was also keen to improve the company's ability to validate therapies advertised by various clinics around the world. ALS TDI researchers would visit medical centers claiming to treat ALS patients and confirm whether the success stories were real. "It's so easy to exploit this group of people that we need to protect them," Jamie says. "I know how terrible the decisions are that people can make when they are desperate about dying and the world is full of charlatans that hurt people. I've watched families give away entire college funds to go do stem cell therapies that I thought were sugar water." But once again, the researchers were forced to make their assessments with little more than a handful of anecdotes. "None of it was quantified," says Jamie.

That was unacceptable. Jamie figured that more than enough patients were trying these therapies that no one should be repeating the same mistakes. Patients needed to start recording their experiences.

And they needed a platform to share those outcomes with others, including statisticians who could analyze the data.

In 2004, Jamie, along with his other brother Ben and a friend, founded PatientsLikeMe. The company launched its flagship ALS community in 2006, and quickly began creating new communities for other diseases. In its first three years, the company added groups for patients with multiple sclerosis, Parkinson's disease, mood disorders, HIV/AIDS, fibromyalgia, chronic fatigue syndrome, and a rare neurological disease called neuromyelitis optica. In 2011, the company opened up its platform to all conditions and grew from just a dozen communities to more than 1,200 in the first year. The database now includes nearly 400,000 members who have shared some 31 million data points about 2,500 different conditions. As the system continues to grow, so will its ability to extract new knowledge about experimental treatments. Jamie and his colleagues have applied these tools to accurately predict the outcomes of clinical trials[14] and to refute the conclusions of others.[15] And in 2012, more than five years after Stephen had passed away, Jamie and his colleagues used the platform to determine whether the stem cell treatment his brother got had helped in any way and whether Jamie had made the right decision in canceling the research program. It hadn't, so he had.

"I think we're entering the era where every one of those treatments can add up to mean something," Jamie says. "And it was almost accidental; like I dreamed it was possible, but the fact that it happened in that way was amazing."

Despite the platform's growth, PatientsLikeMe users still represent a fraction of the global patient community. There remain numerous untapped troves of biomedical data for scientists to mine. Jamie foresees a vast network of clinical research that continuously draws from and contributes to a comprehensive database of patient histories and outcomes. Researchers will be able to use data from all relevant trials to extract information about a disease or drug that could inform the future direction of research. "Suddenly people will wonder why you did experiments any other way," Jamie says. "And we won't know the moment that it died, but the old way will be gone."

On a smaller scale, the idea of using data from the placebo groups of completed clinical trials to bolster analyses of new treatments in development is already being implemented. Neurologist Robert Miller has been collecting such data from ALS trials for fifteen years and has used the database to generate matched controls for recent clinical trials, including the NP001 Phase 2 trial that he helped run at the California Pacific Medical Center. "When you have a small group of patients, with a disease like ALS that has a lot of variation, then you have an imprecise measure of rate of decline," Dr. Miller says. "When you add in historical controls, you get a much more precise placebo rate of decline, and it increases the power of the trial."

Such cases, which already supplement clinical trial data in FDA submissions, could inform a drug's ultimate approval. Dr. Richard Bedlack of Duke ALS Clinic even thinks that one day these historical controls may be used in place of placebo groups in some clinical trials. "We've got thousands of patients that we could use to adequately match every new subject and at least get an idea—is this safe, is this tolerable, is there any kind of borderline efficacy signal that means that this would be worth taking forward into a Phase 3 trial," he says. "I don't think we need a placebo-controlled Phase 2 trial to answer those questions." Pushing the dreaded placebo control off until the very last stage of human trials could reduce the ethical dilemma of giving a fake treatment to fatally ill patients.

In the meantime, DIY medicine is bound to continue, says Jamie, and they might as well be capturing the data patients are willing to share. "There are going to be mistakes and conclusions will be wrong," he said, but potentially biased or incomplete information is better than none at all. He was still staring at that graph of the fourteen ALS patients ingesting sodium chlorite as a substitute for NP001.

Jamie ultimately decided not to share that particular analysis with the patients, but six months later, in October 2012, he openly published a version with data from seventeen patients.[16] Despite the short-lived improvements experienced by some patients, the PatientsLikeMe data pointed to a potentially negative effect of ingesting sodium chlorite. "We have more than 80% confidence that it is worsening patients' progression rate," Jamie and his colleagues wrote.

Jamie still worries that data collected by the PatientsLikeMe platform could be misused. But he believes strongly in patients' rights to make their own treatment decisions, and he wants to help those decisions be as informed as possible. "I don't believe that in America, where the Declaration of Independence has life, liberty, and the pursuit of happiness as a fundamental right, that the regulatory authorities or medical authorities should deny any consenting, understanding patients the ability to do anything that can help them."

Afterword

A subsequent report by ALS Untangled, an organization founded by Dr. Richard Bedlack of the Duke University ALS Clinic to review alternative and off-label treatments, also found that ingesting sodium chlorite doesn't slow ALS progression and may even have a negative effect.[17] NP001, on the other hand, continued to impress. In October 2012, the same month that PatientsLikeMe published its report on sodium chlorite, Neuraltus researchers released its results on the NP001 Phase 2 trial: the high dose of drug notably slowed disease progression, even stopping it altogether in a subset of patients.[18]

Still, it took Neuraltus nearly three years to secure funding for a follow-up trial; it wasn't until July 2015 that the company announced it had raised $1.5 million for a second Phase 2 study. Neuraltus CEO Rich Casey attributes the company's inability to find funds for a full Phase 3 trial to a series of recent failures in the ALS field, including dexpramipexole. Results from the Phase 3 dex trial, released in January 2013, showed that the treatment had failed to slow decline or improve survival.[19] "ALS has been a very bad area for investors," said Casey, who is hoping that the results of the next NP001 Phase 2 trial, which Neuraltus expects to begin this year, will entice further investment in the drug's development.

Eric Valor still lives with his mom and stepdad outside of Santa Cruz, California, and is dating an old friend he reconnected with on Facebook. He continues to be a fierce advocate for the ALS community and for early access to experimental drugs. In 2012, he cofounded the ALS Emergency Treatment Fund (ALS-ETF), which aims to organize early access programs for ALS drugs in development. That August, he was a virtual attendee at a meeting with the FDA, where he and his colleagues made the case that expanded access for patients who don't meet enrollment criteria for clinical trials would not interfere with a drug's continued development, and might even provide data that could inform the design of future trials. ALS-ETF has spoken to multiple companies with ALS drugs in development, and says that its collaborative platform can run a large expanded access program for NP001 at zero cost to the company. Neuraltus says it has no plans to initiate such a program, however.

In 2013, Eric helped launch the SciOpen Research Group, a self-proclaimed "guerrilla biotech" that avoids overhead costs associated with brick-and-mortar aspects of a traditional biotech company. Most recently, he cofounded Hope Now for ALS, which advocates for relaxing the $p < 0.05$ requirement for clinical trials of drugs for fatal diseases, and for patients' access to experimental treatments through the FDA's Accelerated Approval Program. "The struggle continues, with achievement," Eric said. "Hope should never be abandoned, no matter the inevitability."

Author's note

My interest in the ALS community's DIY efforts started in April 2012, with a *Wall Street Journal* article about a group of patients taking a homemade sodium chlorite solution.[20] That summer, I wrote a short piece on the chlorite "trial" for *The Scientist*,[21] where I was—and still am—an editor. But it was clear that seven hundred words did not do the story justice; I needed a whole book to tell the tales of Eric Valor, Ben Harris, and Rob Tison as they spearheaded the sodium chlorite experiments.

I was fortunate to meet both Eric and Ben in the writing of this book, as well as several family members of Eric, Ben, and Rob. I could not have told this story without their support. Thank you for the hours you spent reliving and recounting your experiences with ALS.

While I've focused on the lives of three men, this story is about an entire community. Dozens of other ALS patients and their families were active contributors to the research and discussions surrounding NP001, WF10, and sodium chlorite. It was the very fact that so many contributed their knowledge and data that made this early foray into DIY medicine so exciting.

Notes

1. M. Cudkowicz et al., "The effects of dexpramipexole (KNS-760704) in individuals with amyotrophic lateral sclerosis," *Nature Medicine,* 17: 1652-56, 2011.

2. C. Lomen-Hoerth et al., "Double-blind, placebo controlled safety study of Ritonavir and hydroxyurea in patients with ALS," *Annals of Neurology,* 62 (Suppl. 11): S63, 2007.

3. P. Kaufmann et al., "Phase II trial of CoQ10 for ALS finds insufficient evidence to justify phase III," *Annals of Neurology,* 66: 235-44, 2009.

4. Single-Ascending-Dose Safety/Tolerability of NP001 in Amyotrophic Lateral Sclerosis (ALS), ClinicalTrials.gov Identifier: NCT01091142, 2010.

5. M. McGrath, "Chlorite in the treatment of neurodegenerative disease," US Patent 7105183, Priority date: February 3, 2004.

6. W. Boulanger, A.A. Azhir, "Chlorite formulations and methods of preparation and use thereof," US Patent Application 20120021070, Priority date: December 22, 2005.

7. R. Leuty, "Neuraltus pinning hopes on Lou Gehrig's drug," *San Francisco Business Times,* October 29, 2010.

8. R. Leuty, "Patients enlist in fight against ALS," *San Francisco Business Times,* September 2, 2011.

9. R. Ebert, "Remaking my voice," TED, March 2011.

10. R. Tison, "Persevering on NP001," *Friends4Eric*, January 7, 2012.

11. F. Fornai et al., "Lithium delays progression of amyotrophic lateral sclerosis," *Proceedings of the National Academy of Sciences*, 105: 2052-57, 2008.

12. P. Wicks et al., "A patient-led trial of lithium in ALS using the internet," *Amyotrophic Lateral Sclerosis*, 9 (Suppl. 1): S59, 2008.

13. A. Chiò et al., "Lithium carbonate in amyotrophic lateral sclerosis: Lack of efficacy in a dose-finding trial," *Neurology*, 75: 619-25, 2010; R.G. Miller et al., "Phase II screening trial of lithium carbonate in amyotrophic lateral sclerosis: Examining a more efficient trial design," *Neurology*, 77: 973-79, 2011.

14. P. Wicks et al., "Subjects no more: What happens when trial participants realize they hold the power?" *BMJ*, 348: g368, 2014.

15. P. Wicks et al., "Accelerated clinical discovery using self-reported patient data collected online and a patient-matching algorithm," *Nature Biotechnology*, 29: 411-14, 2011.

16. J. Heywood et al., "Waiting for $p < 0.05$," figshare, 2012.

17. The ALSUntangled Group, "ALSUntangled No. 19: Sodium chlorite," *Amyotrophic Lateral Sclerosis and Frontotemporal Degeneration*, 14: 236-38, 2013.

18. Later published as R.G. Miller et al., "Randomized Phase 2 trial of NP001, a novel immune regulator," *Neurology: Neuroimmunology & Neuroinflammation*, 2: e100, 2015.

19. Later published as M.E. Cudkowicz et al., "Dexpramipexole versus placebo for patients with amyotrophic lateral sclerosis (EMPOWER): A randomised, double-blind, Phase 3 trial," *The Lancet Neurology*, 12: 1059-67, 2013.

20. A.D. Marcus, "Frustrated ALS patients concoct their own drug," *The Wall Street Journal*, April 15, 2012.

21. J. Akst, "Medical Mavericks," *The Scientist*, July 1, 2012.